Strive to Thrive *Today*

Getting Better...One Day At A Time

Bill Durkin

Copyright© 2013 Bill Durkins
Published by One Positive Place Inc.
760 Village Center Drive, Suite 210
Burr Ridge, Illinois 60527

Design by Brian Frantz

All rights reserved. No portion of this publication may be reproduced,
stored in a retrieval system or transmitted in any form by any means —
except for brief quotations in printed reviews — without the prior
written permission of the publisher.

Images by: ShutterStock images
ISBN 978-0-9893733-0-2
01 WOZ 13

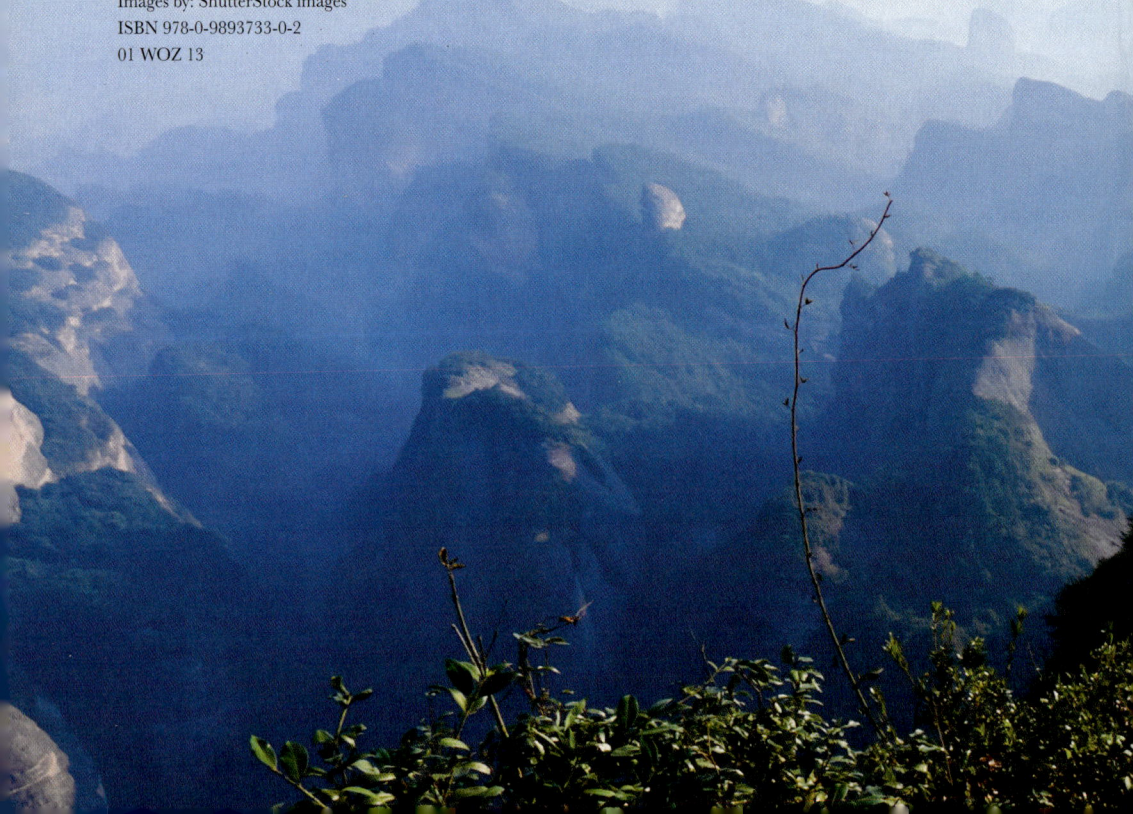

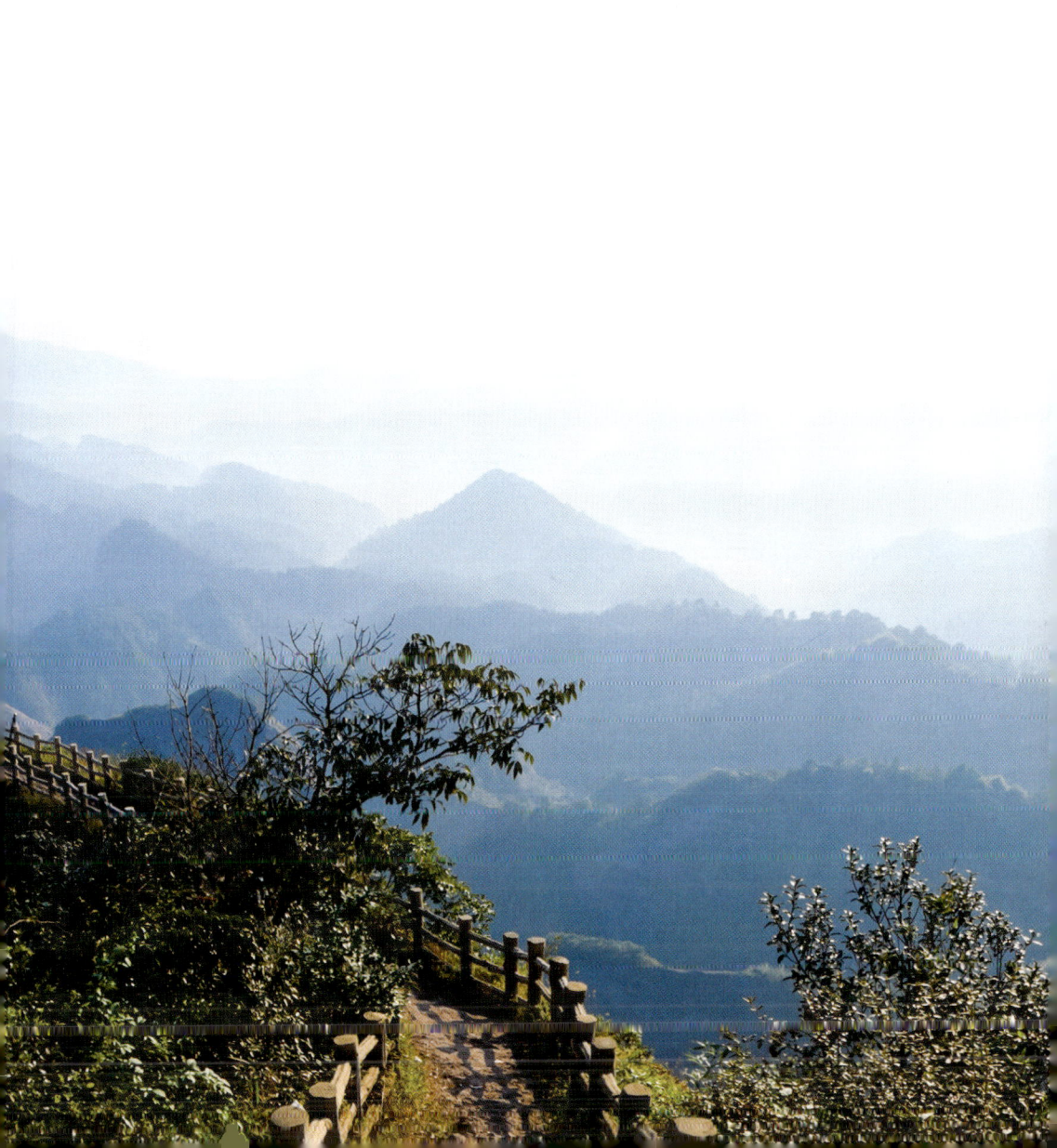

Dedication

To my beautiful wife Joan and two remarkable boys, Billy and Bobby, thank you for your unconditional love, encouragement and inspiration. I thank God every day that you are in my life.

To my brother Bob, thank you for showing me how to overcome adversity, move forward one day at a time and have fun while serving others. You have been and will continue to be a positive influence in my life.

To my Mother, Aunt and Sister, thank you for all your love and prayers and for teaching me the importance of having a strong relationship with God and my family.

And to…

My dad, Coach Bill Durkin. Thank you for showing me and all your students and players how to thrive. You brought out the best in all of us!

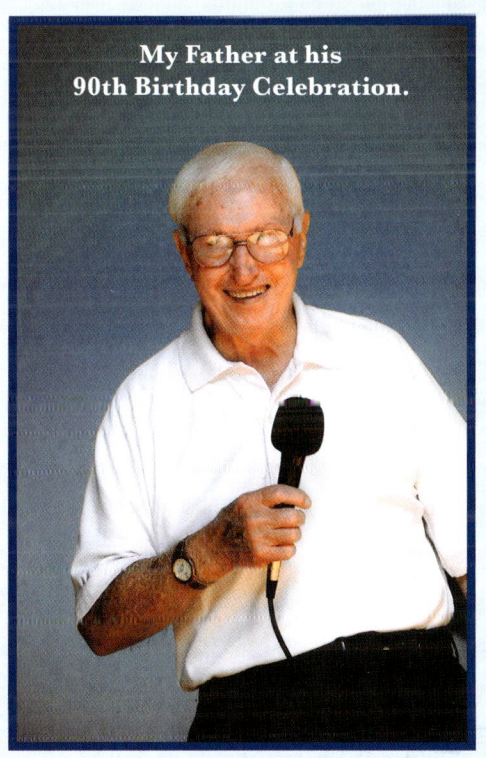

April 22, 1922 — November 19, 2012

Contents

Introduction....10

Accept What You Cannot Change....12

Change What You Can....24

Acquire Wisdom To Know The Difference....64

Get Better...One Day At A Time....84

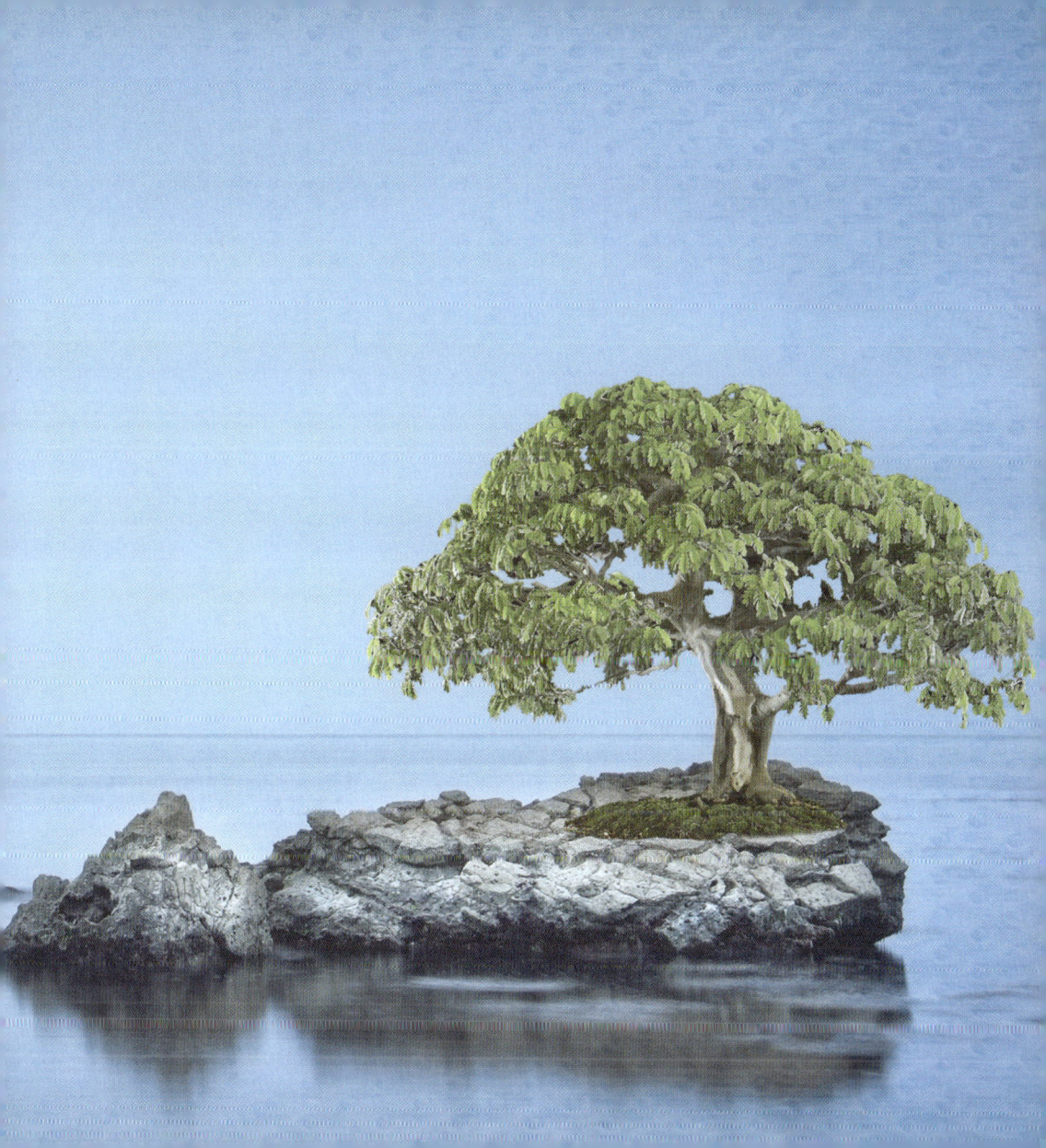

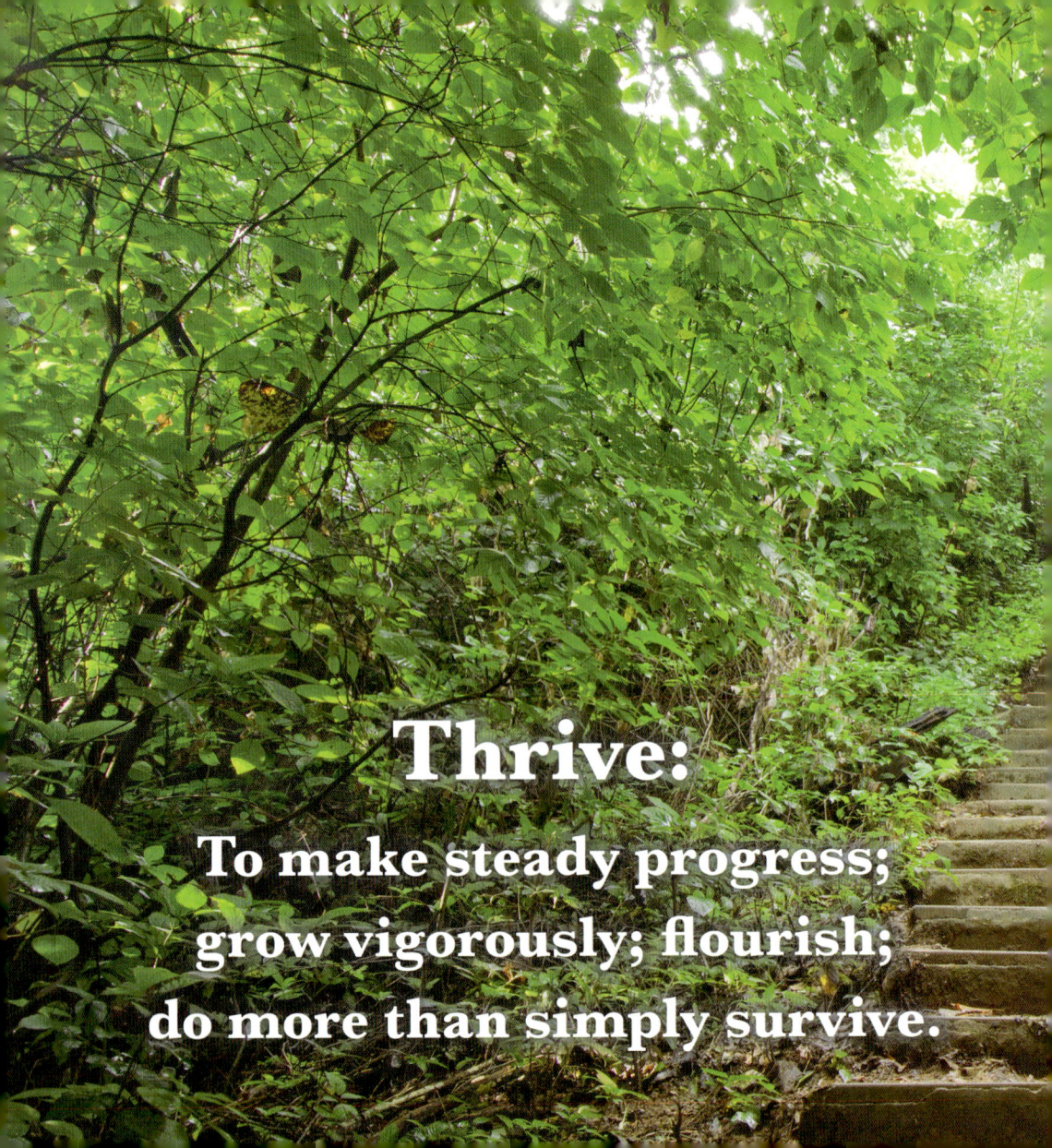

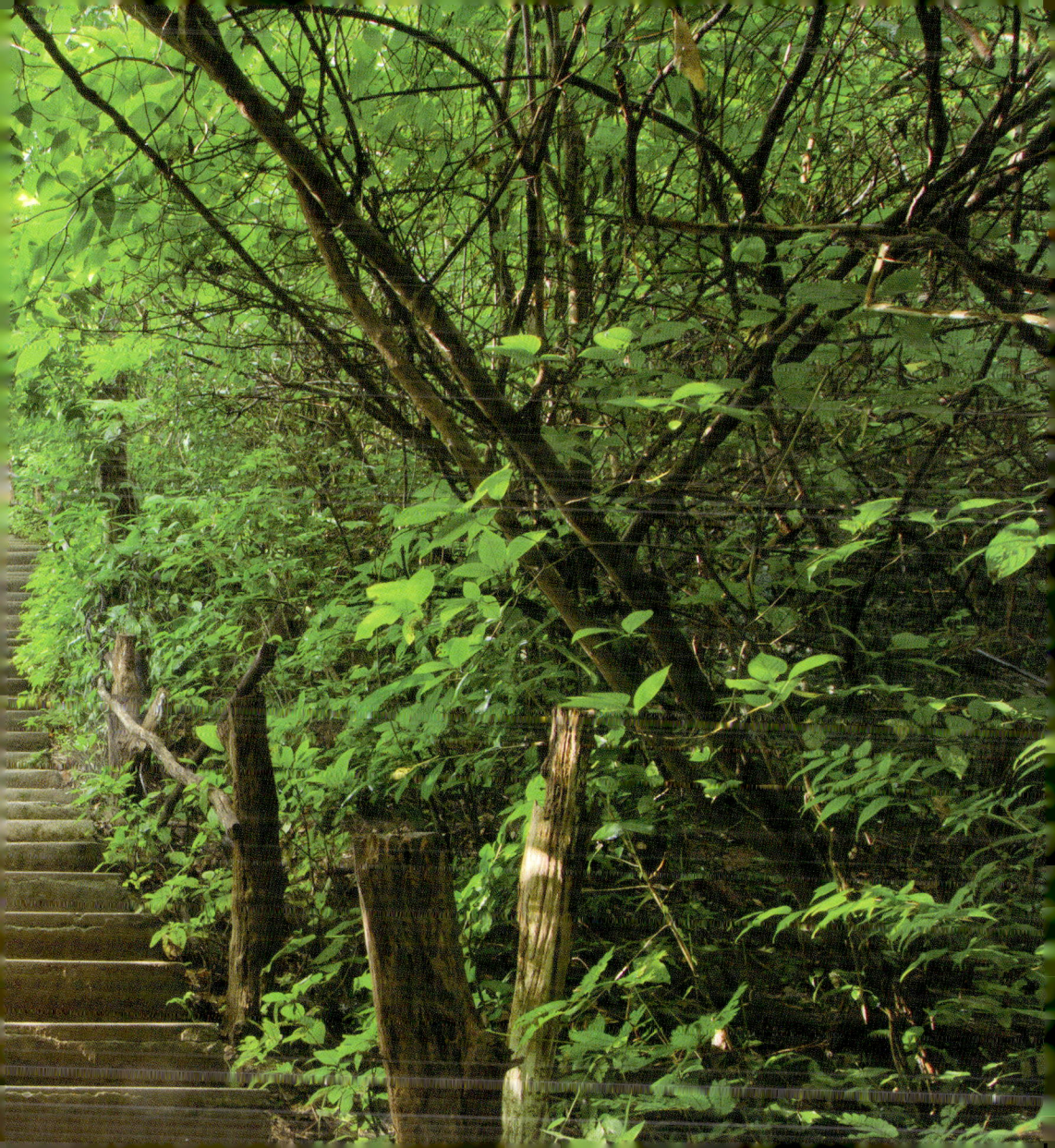

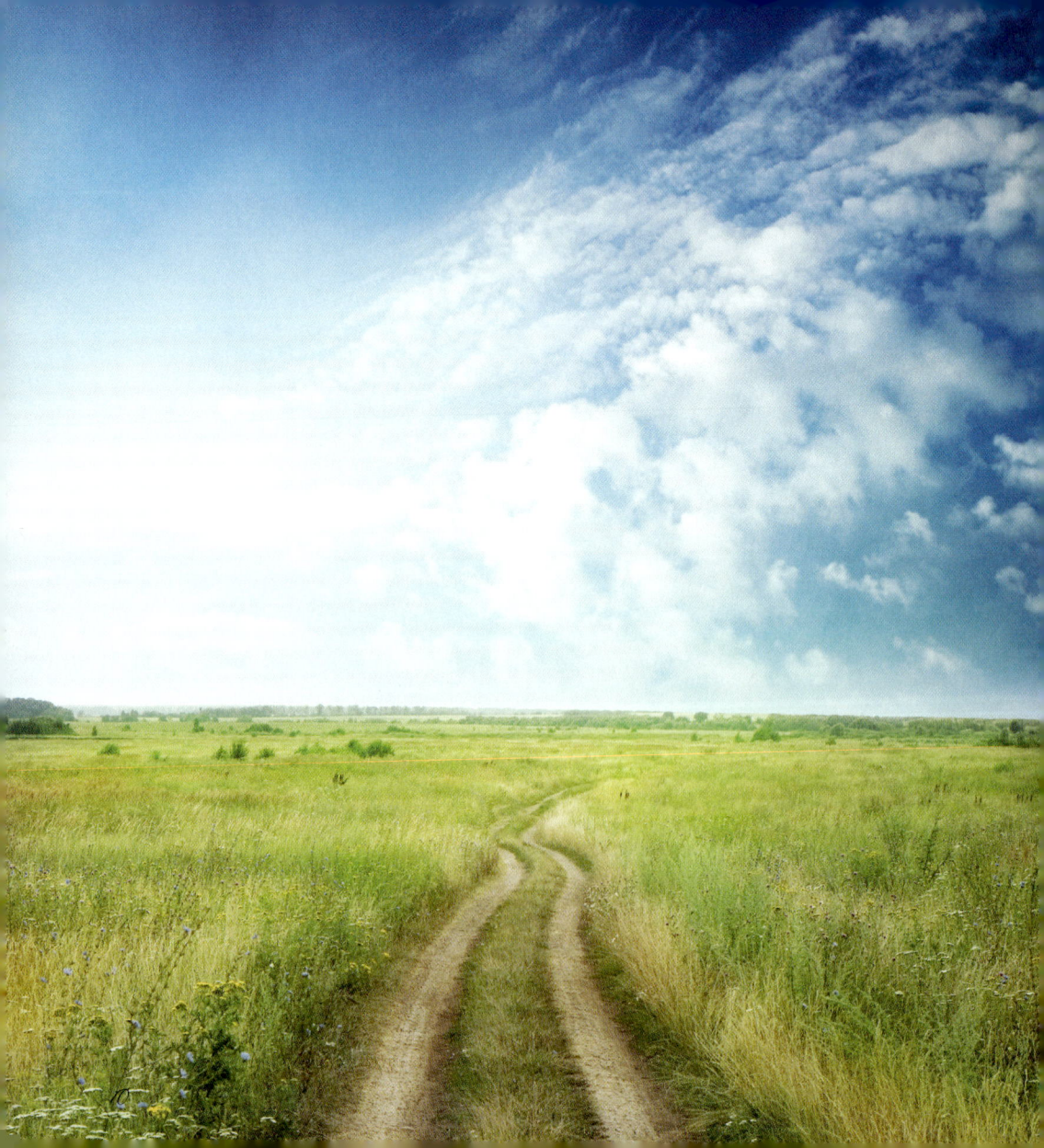

Introduction

Being in the hospital is difficult for anyone. You may feel that your life, as well as your health, are out of your control. But, even in the midst of illness and pain, it is still possible to take charge of your own well-being…and **Strive to Thrive Today!**

The threshold for pain is unique to each one of us. So are the actions we take. How do you determine when to fight and when to let go? When to ask for help and when to help others? When simply surviving should be your goal or when it's time to thrive? Our choices are intensely personal.

But, regardless of how you are feeling, know that you have a choice about how to view your circumstances.

Viktor Frankl, a Holocaust survivor and author of *"Man's Search for Meaning"* said it best, "Everything can be taken from a man but one thing: the last of human freedoms - to choose one's attitude in any given set of circumstances, to choose one's own way."

It is my hope that the stories and information I share will help you navigate and come to terms with your pain and perhaps even encourage you to use your experience and unique strength to inspire others to thrive.

Accept What You Cannot Change

Accept What You Cannot Change

I'd like to explain a little of my personal challenge with pain and injury and how one simple sentence made all the difference in my ability to thrive in spite of the suffering I was experiencing.

I spent my life attempting to avoid pain, making every effort to safeguard myself from the potential of physical discomfort. I worked out regularly, ate vegetarian meals, and attended three different churches. I somehow believed that if I just managed to live right, nothing would go wrong.

When I turned 45, my fixation on health and fitness accelerated. I hired a personal trainer. She convinced me the key to fitness in my forties was weight training. Within minutes of our second session, I managed to induce what I had spent a lifetime trying to avoid: excruciating pain. I had herniated a disk in my back, my sciatic nerve was damaged, and I could no longer walk, sit or lie down without extreme discomfort.

I couldn't work and was losing money every month. I loved playing basketball, golf and doing triathlons, but I had to give all that up. I was in my mid-forties and still single. My Irish Catholic mother and aunt rarely left their prayer chairs asking God to give me a better back and a bride. I felt my spirit was beyond renewal.

One day, while in the depth of my darkness and feeling very sorry for myself, I noticed *"The Serenity Prayer"* I had on a plaque in my office.

The Serenity Prayer

God grant me the serenity

to accept the things I cannot change,

courage to change the things I can,

and wisdom to know the difference.

It had been there for years, but I had never really concentrated on the entire message. My efforts had always been directed toward finding the courage to change my circumstances. It didn't occur to me that I should also develop the ability to accept the things I couldn't change.

Accept What You Cannot Change

Acceptance and Serenity

When I first thought about the possibility of accepting my life would be different, I felt like a quitter. I told myself I should never give up on getting my old life back. I begged, pleaded, bargained and I still suffered physically, spiritually and financially. When I ultimately accepted my situation, my back pain and financial situation remained the same, but my emotional pain turned to peace.

Twelve months after my accident I had successful back surgery. My recovery wasn't easy or fast and my financial problems continued to climb because I was unable to work for several months after the operation. To make matters worse, my insurance company found a loophole in my policy and informed me that they were not going to pay my medical bills.

In spite of everything that was happening, I was amazed how easy it was for me to renew my spirit by ***accepting the things I could not change.*019**

Today, I'm happily married to a wonderful woman and am the father of two remarkable boys. I don't believe I would be a husband or a dad today if I didn't experience the suffering and insights that came as a result of my back injury. I approach my family and work with peace and passion. Life still has its ups and downs, but I am no longer worried about things outside my control.

As a result of my injury, I changed my priorities and the way I spent my time. I would never have believed it the day I damaged my back, but getting hurt changed my life for the better.

The Positive Part of Pain

When an unexpected illness or debilitating medical problem is approached rather than avoided, the results can be enlightening and empowering. Anyone who has taken on the challenge of driving during a Midwestern winter has likely experienced the overpowering feeling of helplessness when the car suddenly veers on an icy highway. The vehicle slides. You immediately grasp the wheel and attempt to steer. The illusion of control is soon replaced by reality; you're merely hanging on with little recourse but to go along for the ride. The same can occur with suffering.

Our inclination as human beings is to steer our destinies with both hands on the wheel, but events beyond our control quickly remind us that life cannot be managed. When pain and suffering are thrust upon us, loss of control is one of the most powerful feelings people experience.

It's natural to feel fearful during an illness. There's uncertainty of its impact on your future, your plans and your overall quality of life. With chronic pain, what was once predictable becomes contingent upon how you're feeling. Whether you take a vacation, go to work or simply interact with others depends on whether or not the pain takes over at any given moment.

Many people, when returning home from the hospital perceive they have become a strain on others. Feeling much like an uninvited guest, they begin to believe they are a burden. In spite of the prevailing fears and doubts, tragedy can bring us closer to our loved ones and teach us some important life lessons. However, we do have to learn to stay optimistic and choose to accept what cannot be changed. There is a positive side to pain but you have to be willing to create it.

"We waste so much energy fighting the nature of life. Accept the nature of life and surrender to it. Surrender is not about doing nothing; it is about doing the right things.

When you surrender to the illness, you continue to receive your treatments and do all the other work of healing. But while you are working, you are saying, 'Thy will be done' and not 'My will be done.' Surrender the pain, fear and worries and you'll be able to keep love, hope and joy in your life."

–Dr. Bernie Siegel

Sleep on the Side of the Pain

In the weeks after my surgery, I struggled to rest at night and assumed that I should try to sleep on the opposite side of the pain. I just couldn't get comfortable. During my routine exam, I asked my doctor for his advice.

I was surprised and somewhat skeptical when my physician instructed me to "sleep on the side of the pain." In effect, I was asked to move closer to the physical source of anguish and embrace the pain.

My instincts advised me to flee in the opposite direction, but instead I learned a useful lesson. As normal as it is to curse the loss that can come from suffering, experiencing the pain while staying positive provides opportunities for unforeseen gains.

Being optimistic will not automatically turn pain to pleasure or fix all our problems. But it will help us accept the things we cannot change. When accepted and embraced, suffering presents an opportunity for renewal, allowing us to re-evaluate, shift priorities, simplify our lives, and clarify our values. When we accept our vulnerability during an illness, we realize that while much has been taken away, it is still possible to sustain a meaningful life and create new opportunities for happiness.

As our days turn into years, we become aware that illness or even natural disasters reinforce the reality that life is beyond our control. We cannot completely safeguard ourselves from every impending danger. Sickness is an inevitable deterioration that occurs in our bodies, but often it's difficult to view it as a natural process.

When we can learn to accept that health is not a birthright ... wellness is not achieved by a quick fix ... and illness is a natural part of life, acceptance can make us stronger. We can't control all the things that happen to us, but we can reinvent our response. We can make positive choices…we can choose to accept what can't be changed and still **Strive to Thrive Today!**

When people are able to accept the things in their lives that they can't control—from illness to job loss to relationship disappointment—it can be empowering.

As part of our journey towards acceptance, we have the opportunity to become more humble, to develop a greater need to serve others, to

Accept What You Cannot Change

find meaningful new work, to grow stronger in our faith and closer to those we love. It's hardly a coincidence that so many of the great works of art, literature, film and music have been produced when the artists were either emerging from or in the midst of sickness or suffering. It can infuse us with a renewed sense of passion and purpose.

My own personal story of pain and recovery provided unanticipated opportunities to take a closer look at the quality of my life. Since my injury, I am more committed to spending time with family and close friends…to being a positive influence on the people I meet…to doing my best to grow vigorously and make steady progress toward meaningful goals each day.

When the pace of life involuntarily slows, it can be surprising what comes into focus. While suffering is certainly not the type of challenge any of us want, the lessons learned while in pain are practical, potent and ultimately inspiring. Looking for the positive potential in problems gives us a chance to create value from them, if we decide to accept what cannot be changed.

"Acceptance means embracing what is, rather than wishing for what is not. When we accept difficult realities, we are able to discover whatever positive feelings and experiences may be possible in that situation. We find ourselves more at peace and able to experience life more deeply. Even so, acceptance must be guided by discernment – learning how to tell the difference between what we can change and what we cannot."

–Wisdom Commons   www.wisdomcommons.org

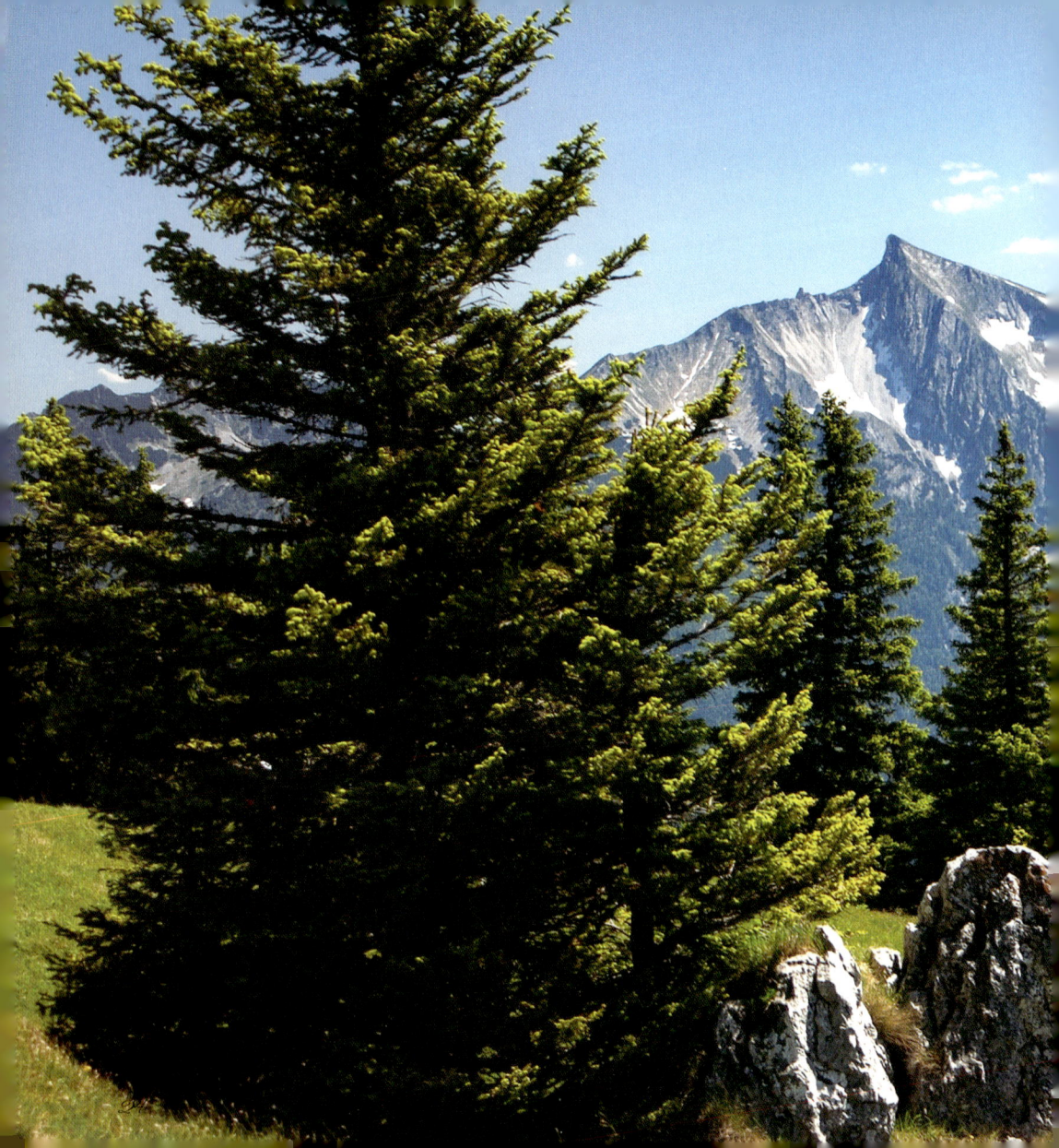

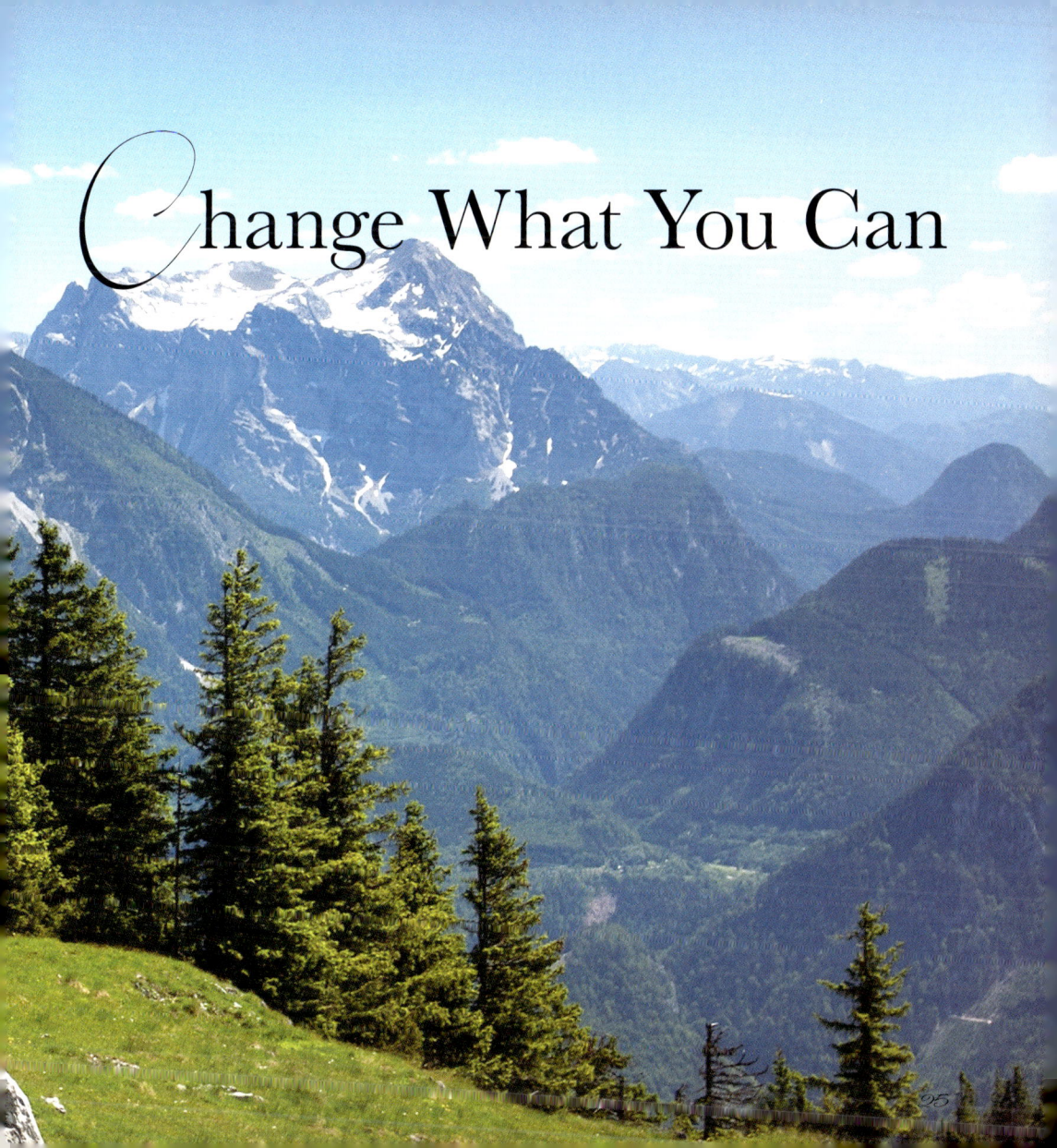

Change What You Can

It's not surprising that we can feel at our most vulnerable when facing the unknowns of being hospitalized. Anxiety comes from feeling out of control. *What will the tests reveal? When will I see my doctor? Will I be able to manage my pain after surgery? How soon can I go home? Who will be there with support through my recovery?*

The hospital experience can be an overpowering source of angst because so much seems out of our hands. Yet as patients, we can identify those situations within our control and make positive choices.

When we take positive action daily, it can reduce conflict and anxiety, keep our spirits up when life gets us down and ultimately contribute to our healing and recovery.

How can you start to shift the focus from feelings of distress to areas within your control? One helpful approach is to think differently about what it means to be a patient.

You might think being in the hospital is a passive experience—you sit back and let the medical professionals tell you what to do while you watch TV, read magazines and hope for the best. But when you take this approach, you surrender responsibility for your recovery. You relinquish your role as an active participant in your own health and healing.

When you choose to be a positive partner in your recovery, the results can have a dramatic impact spiritually, emotionally and physically—for yourself and the people committed to caring for you.

Occasionally I caught myself focusing on negative thoughts while in the hospital. I think all patients do from time to time. The problem isn't the thought, it's how much time you allow yourself to spend on negativity. As you move from surviving to thriving, learn to fill your mind with positive stories.

Thinking about W. Mitchell always helped me get back on the positive path. Years after he was in a fiery motorcycle accident and a paralyzing plane crash, he told me how he learned to take responsibility for the new challenges in his life. He decided to live by the philosophy, "It's not what happens to you. It's what you do about it." Mitchell proved to himself and others that he could create something positive out of adversity. One statement he made really inspired me: *"Before I was paralyzed, there were 10,000 things I could do. Now there are 9,000. I can either dwell on the 1,000 I've lost or focus on the 9,000 I have left."* Whenever I start thinking about what I can't do, I tell myself..."If Mitchell can think positive thoughts, so can I." I believe the same is true for you.

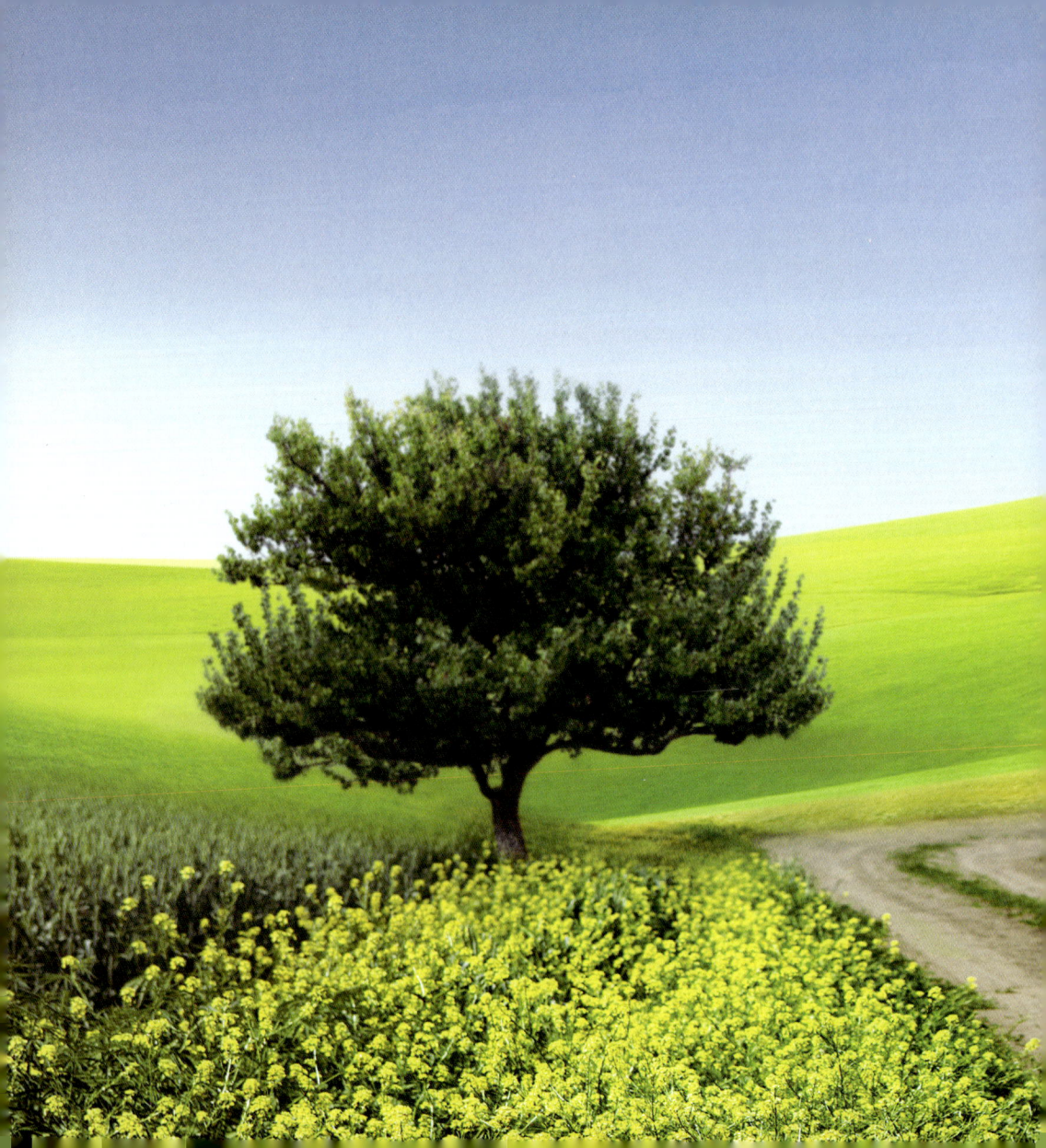

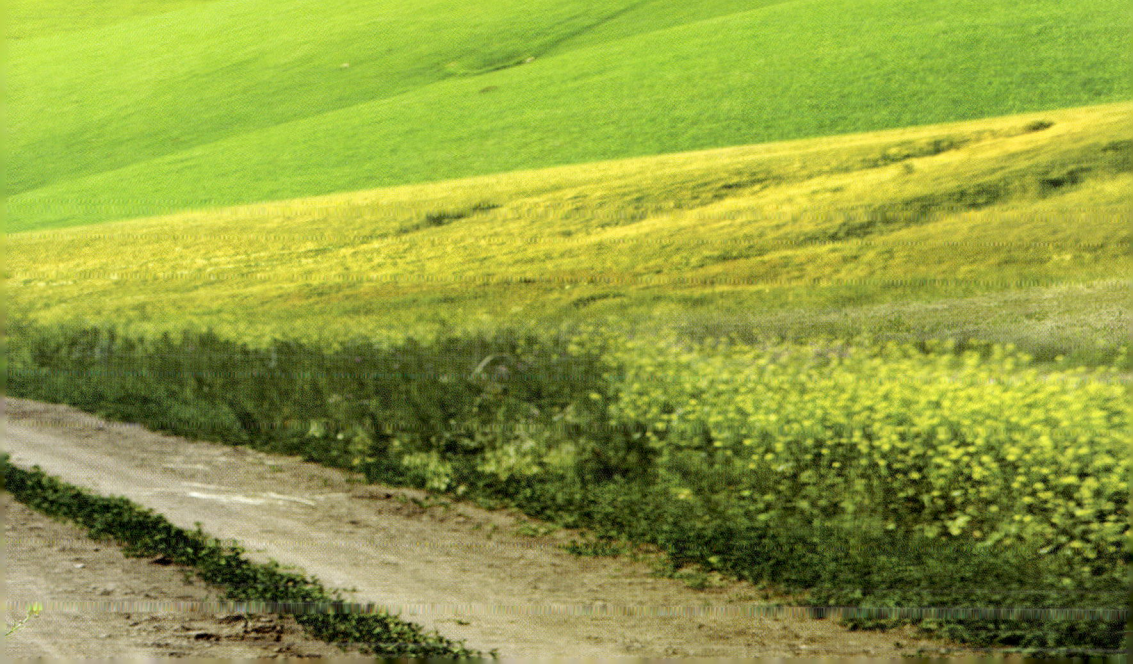

But, simply repeating positive sayings will not make a meaningful difference in the quality of your life when you are dealing with pain and suffering. You have to train yourself to have an authentically positive point of view.

Unfortunately, you don't have to do anything to be negative. The world will gladly help you reach that goal without any effort on your part. Being optimistic, on the other hand, requires work. However, if you decide to develop the daily discipline of planting positive seeds in your mind, you will strengthen your positivity muscles, build resilience and thrive.

Barbara Fredrickson, Ph.D., and distinguished Professor of Psychology at the University of North Carolina, and winner of numerous honors for her research on positive emotions and mental health, identifies six important scientific facts about positivity.

1. ***Positivity Feels Good.*** Focusing on the positive makes you feel better.

2. ***Positivity Broadens Minds.*** Being positive opens your mind and expands your ability to see more of what's positive in your world.

3. ***Positivity Builds Resources.*** Focusing on the positive over time builds mental strength. You become stronger and wiser. Positivity helps you grow vigorously and thrive.

4. **_Positivity Fuels Resilience._** When negativity strikes you down, positivity stops your fall and helps you bounce back.

5. **_Positivity Ratios Above 3 Positives to 1 Negative Forecast Flourishing._** This refers to creating at least three positive thoughts for each negative one. Most people never go above 2-1. At this level, you are able to survive but not thrive. 3-1 is the tipping point for you to start to flourish and move to a much higher quality of life.

6. **_People Can Raise Their Positivity Ratios._** Through your own efforts, you can raise your positivity ratio and move from surviving to thriving. We all have more control over our thoughts than we realize.

Increasing your self-talk awareness is a good way to start raising your Positivity Ratio. We talk to ourselves all day long and these unspoken thoughts are often negative. Pessimistic patients have a tendency to expect the worst when it comes to their recovery. While there are some situations where you can benefit from looking at the downside of a situation, improving the quality of your health is not one of them.

Negative thoughts don't just come one at a time. They come in large numbers like waves crashing on a shore. At first they have little impact on us, but soon our mind creates a hurricane of negativity and we get crushed by unhealthy feelings of anxiety and fear.

Many people get angry with themselves when they enter the hospital and start turning their negativity and criticism inward. Let me ask you…"If someone talked to you the way you're talking to yourself, how long would you hang around with them?" If you want to thrive, you have to be your own best friend, in and out of the hospital.

The moment you become aware of a negative thought, you can choose to change your focus. Make a decision right now that you are going to fill your mind with positivity during your healing process. Everything you say to yourself matters, so start having more positive conversations. Remember the 3-1 ratio. Create at least 3 positive thoughts for every negative idea that enters your mind.

You also have to continually monitor your Positivity, just like your nurses frequently assess your pain. Why do medical professionals keep asking you about your pain? Because when your caregivers are aware of your pain level, they can do a much better job of treating you properly. The same is true when it comes to managing your positivity.

The Bible says in Philippians 4:8 *"Whatever is true, whatever is noble, whatever is right, whatever is pure, whatever is lovely, whatever is admirable, whatever is excellent, or worthy of praise, think on these things."* That's good advice for all of us.

"By making more moments glisten with positivity, you make the choice of a lifetime: you choose the upward spiral that leads to your best future – and to our best world."
–Barbara Fredrickson, PhD

Change What You Can

"My friends, love is better than anger. Hope is better than fear. Optimism is better than despair. So let us be loving, hopeful and optimistic. And we'll change the world."

—Jack Layton

Where are you right now on the Positivity Scale?

| 0 | 2 | 4 | 6 | 8 | 10 |

0 .... Always Positive

2 .... Mostly Positive

4 .... A little more Positive than Negative

6 .... A little more Negative than Positive

8 .... Mostly Negative

10 .... Always Negative

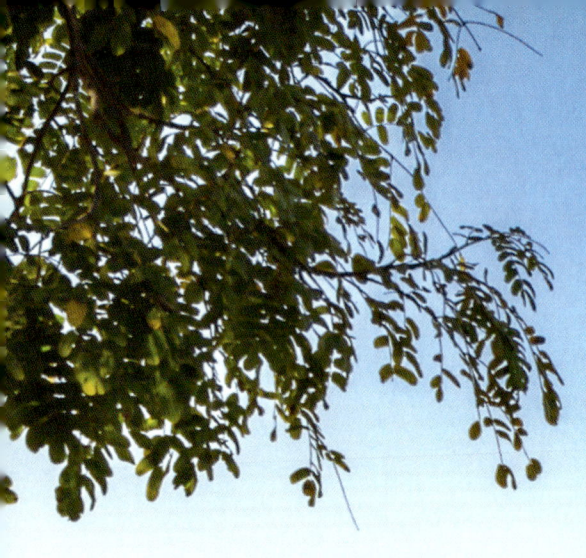

I'm not denying the fact that pain and suffering are part of living. I know bad things happen to good people, but positive people make the best out of challenging situations. Positive people are creators not critics.

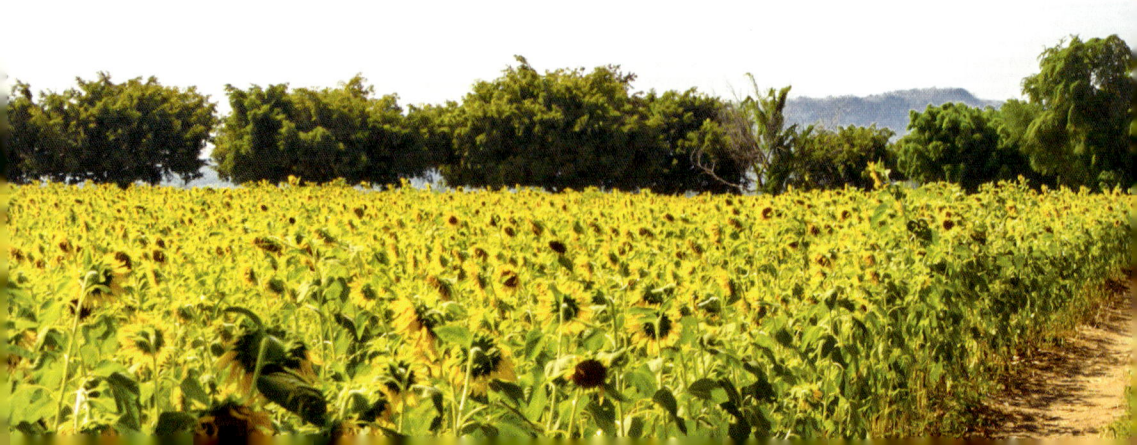

Our homes, hospitals, schools, places of work and worship are filled with remarkable people who are making a positive difference in the lives of others. Listen to their stories. Don't let the local and national television stations, news media, and even some family and friends bombard you with a daily dose of negativity. The quality of your life will dramatically improve when you break the habit of listening to negative information.

Yes it's true that bad news sells, but you don't have to buy it. Start collecting and sharing information that inspires positive emotions. Decide today that you are going to look for the good in yourself and others. When you learn to shed a little light during your darkest days, everyone's life gets brighter.

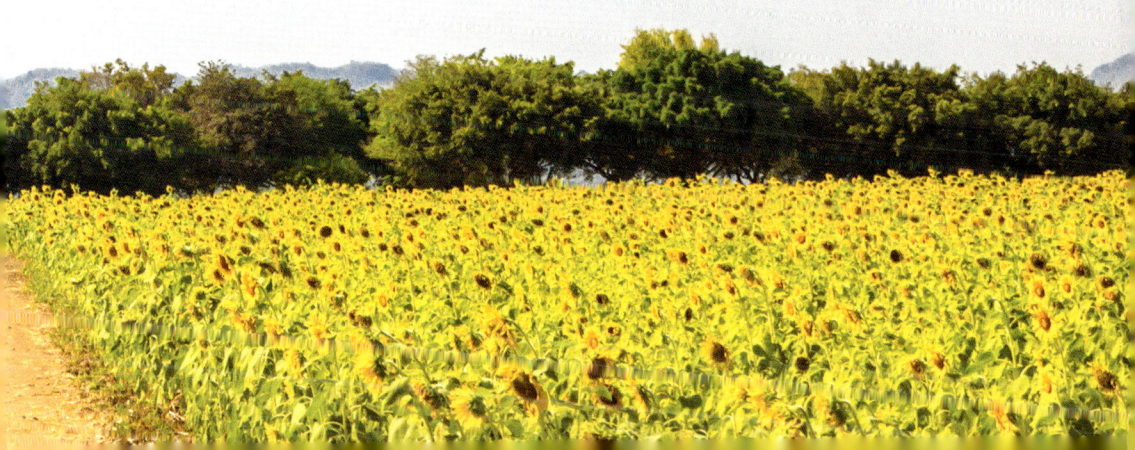

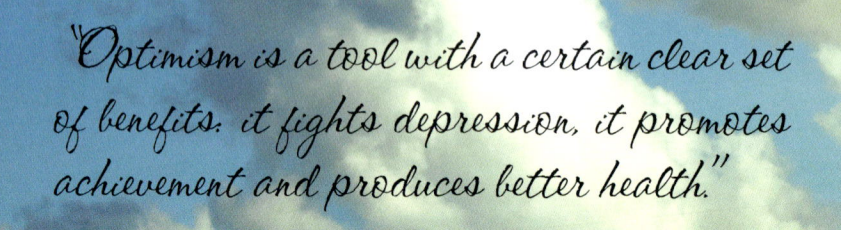

"Optimism is a tool with a certain clear set of benefits: it fights depression, it promotes achievement and produces better health."

–Martin Seligman

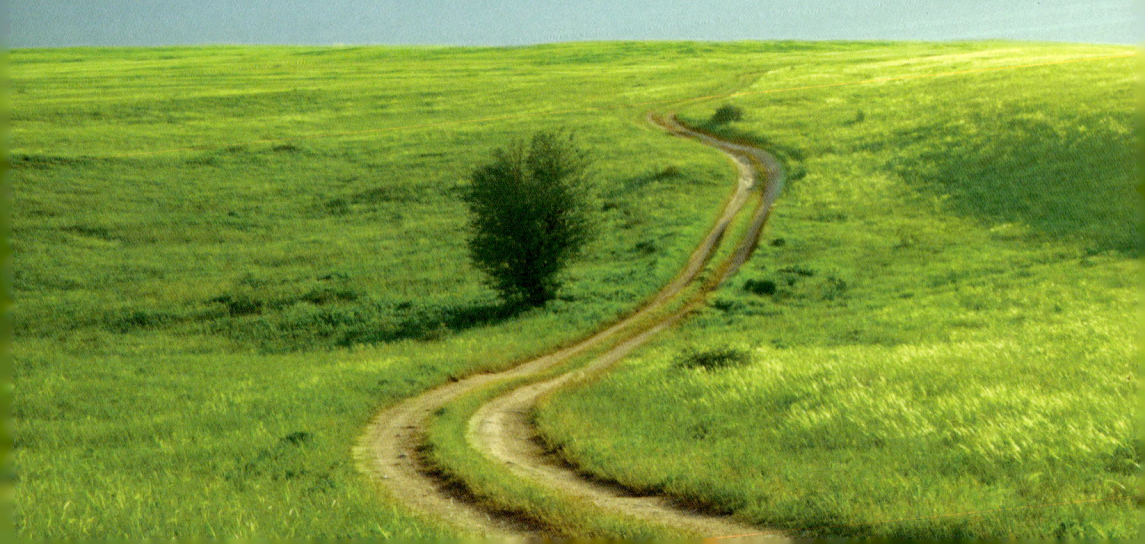

Good News For A Change

The Mayo Clinic reports a number of health benefits associated with optimism, including a reduced risk of death from cardiovascular problems, less depression, and an increased life span. While researchers are not entirely clear on why positive thinking benefits health, one theory suggests a positive outlook enables you to cope better with stressful situations, which reduces the harmful health effects of stress on your body.

Take Positive Action Today

An excellent way to develop optimism and accelerate your recovery is by taking positive action every day. In fact, it's easier to act your way into positive thinking than it is to think your way into positive action.

Start by rewriting the antiquated patient handbook from the 1950s. Instead of waiting for the healing to begin, steer your recovery with a positive action strategy. Whether you were admitted to the hospital because of an illness or injury, or have planned a hospital stay for surgery or testing, make a commitment to take the positive approach during your healing process.

The following Positive Action Plan for Patients can help you improve the quality of your life in and out of the hospital. <u>Review the Positive Actions on pages 43-60</u>, decide what ideas might work for you and get into action.

The Positive Action Plan for Patients

For a more detailed description of these 10 Positive Actions,

please visit:

www.*strivetothrivetoday*.com

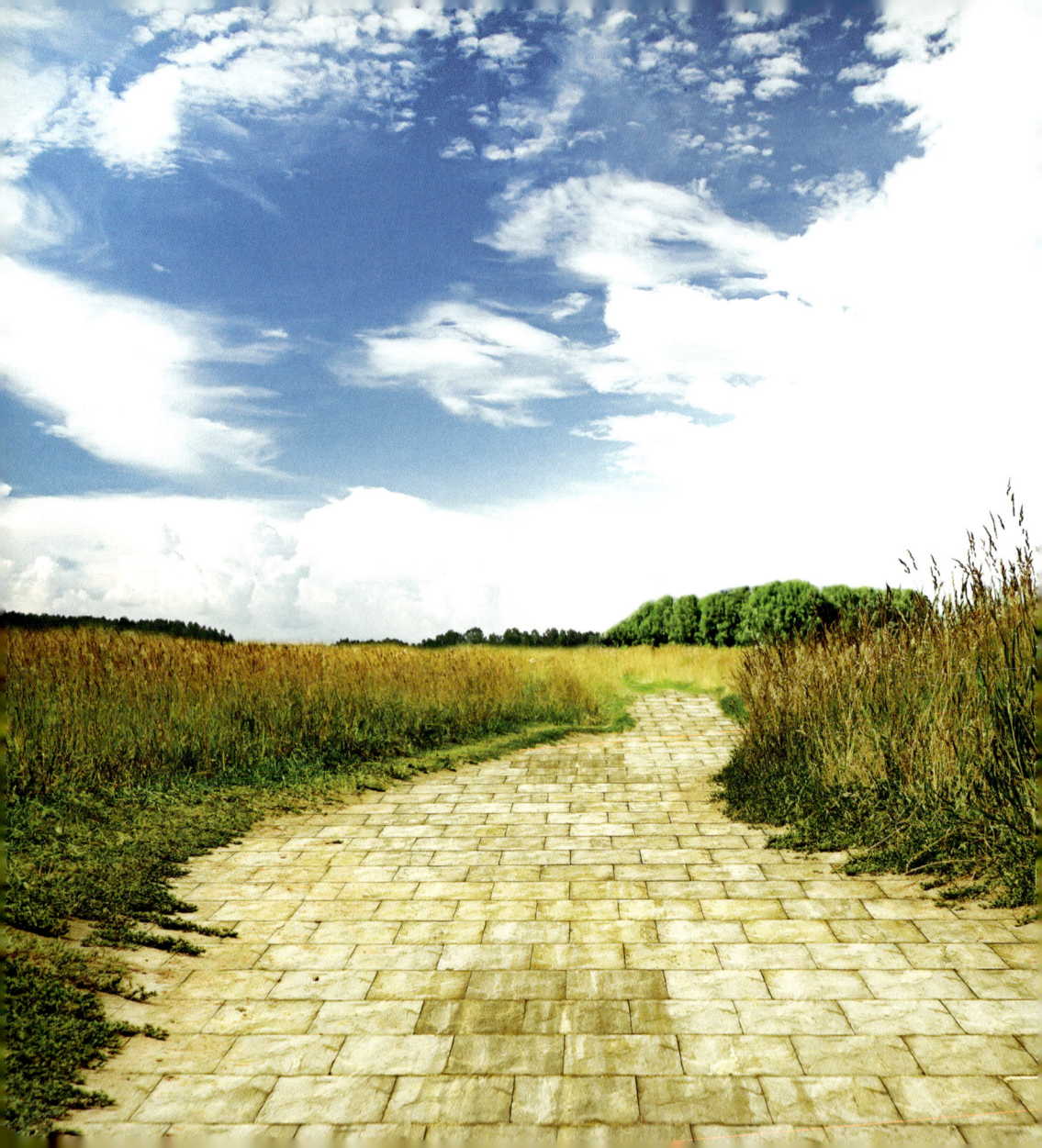

#1 Take an active role in your health.

Be a Positive Participant in your care. Make the commitment to partner with your physicians, nurses and caregivers in the healing process. Know about your treatment and medication plans after you leave the hospital. Working together with your caregivers while in the hospital, and for at least 30 days after you leave, is the best way to improve the quality of your health.

A recent report from The Robert Wood Johnson Foundation called, *"Care About Your Care"* found more than 1 million Americans wind up back in the hospital only weeks after being discharged for reasons that could have been prevented. The most common cause for avoidable readmissions is that patients don't understand their discharge instructions. Take personal responsibility for making sure you or someone you know completely understands what you need to do when you leave the hospital.

Be the positive core of your health care team. ***Strive to Thrive Today!***

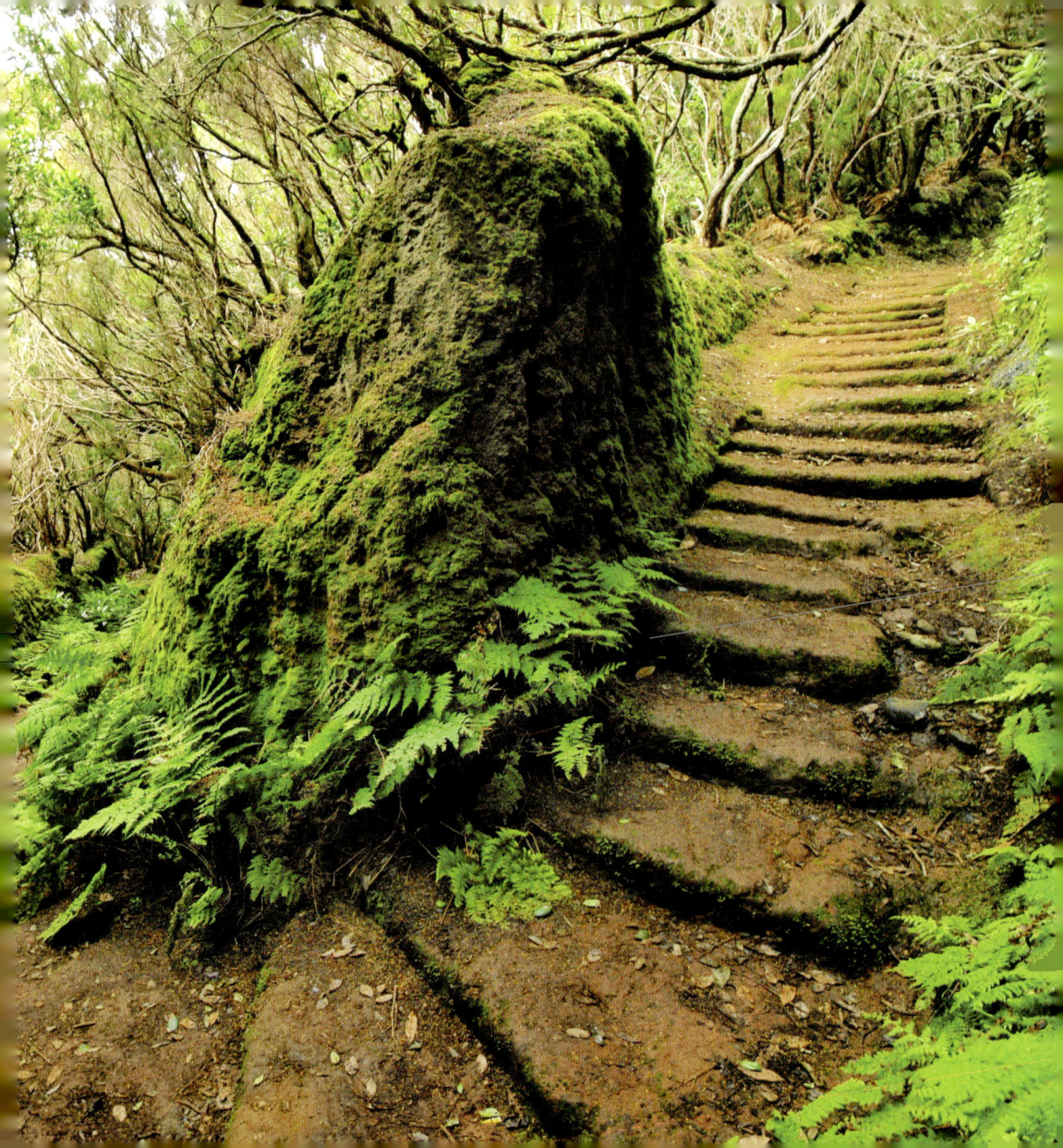

#2

Listen and ask questions.

Make the most of your interactions with your care team. Allow your doctors and nurses to explain your diagnosis and treatment. Listen without interrupting and then summarize your understanding of what you heard. If you don't comprehend something, ask for clarification. If you need more information, schedule another meeting and prepare a list of questions you want answered. When it's your turn to share, be as clear and concise as possible. If your doctor or nurse interrupts you, politely ask them to listen a little longer. Make good communication a priority.

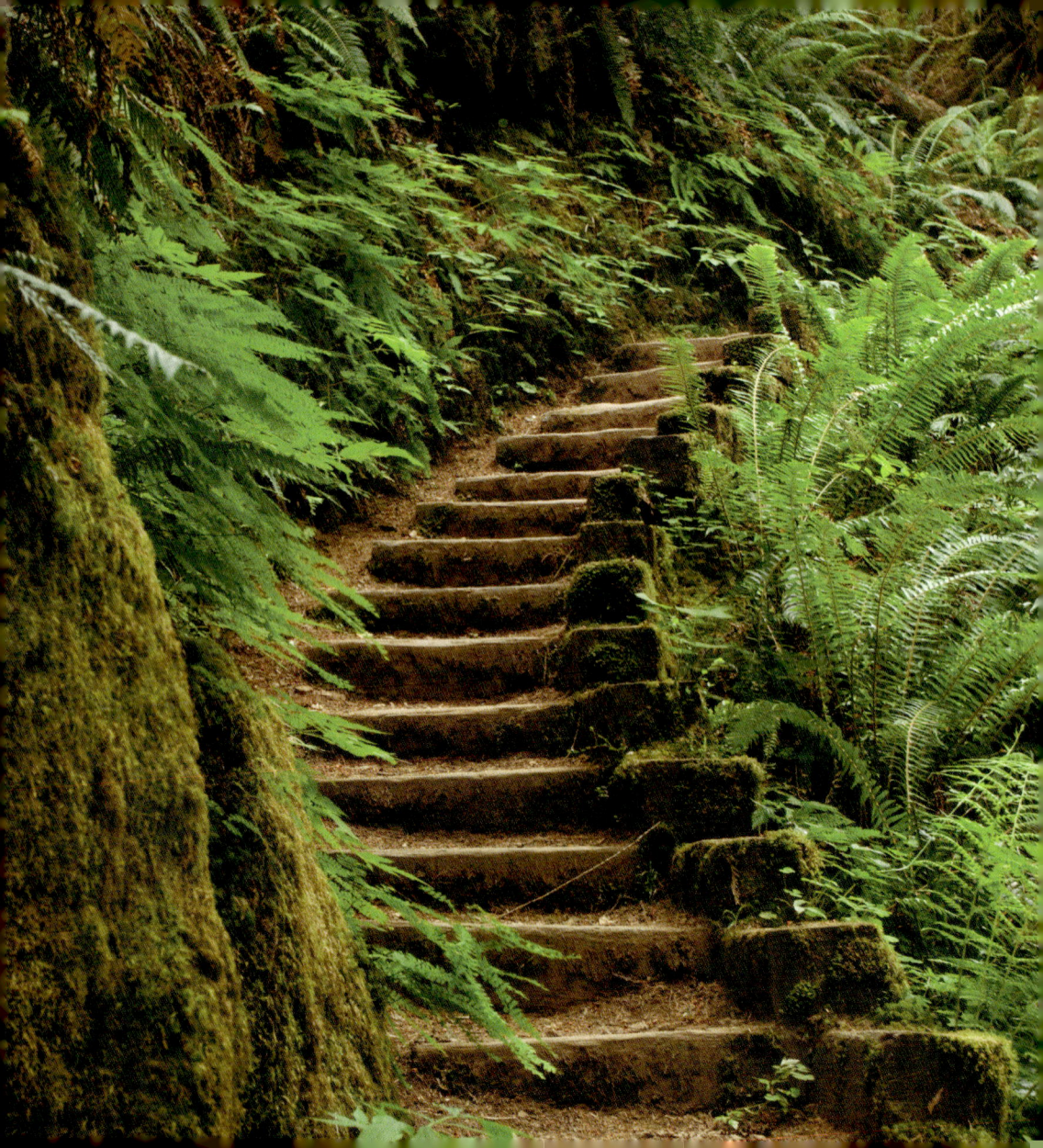

#3

Keep a medical notebook and personal journal.

Be prepared when consulting with your physicians and nurses. Use a bedside notebook to jot down medical questions and concerns. Take notes to remember important information and instructions. Use a personal journal to express your thoughts and feelings to help you through the stages of your physical and emotional recovery. If you can't write, use a recorder.

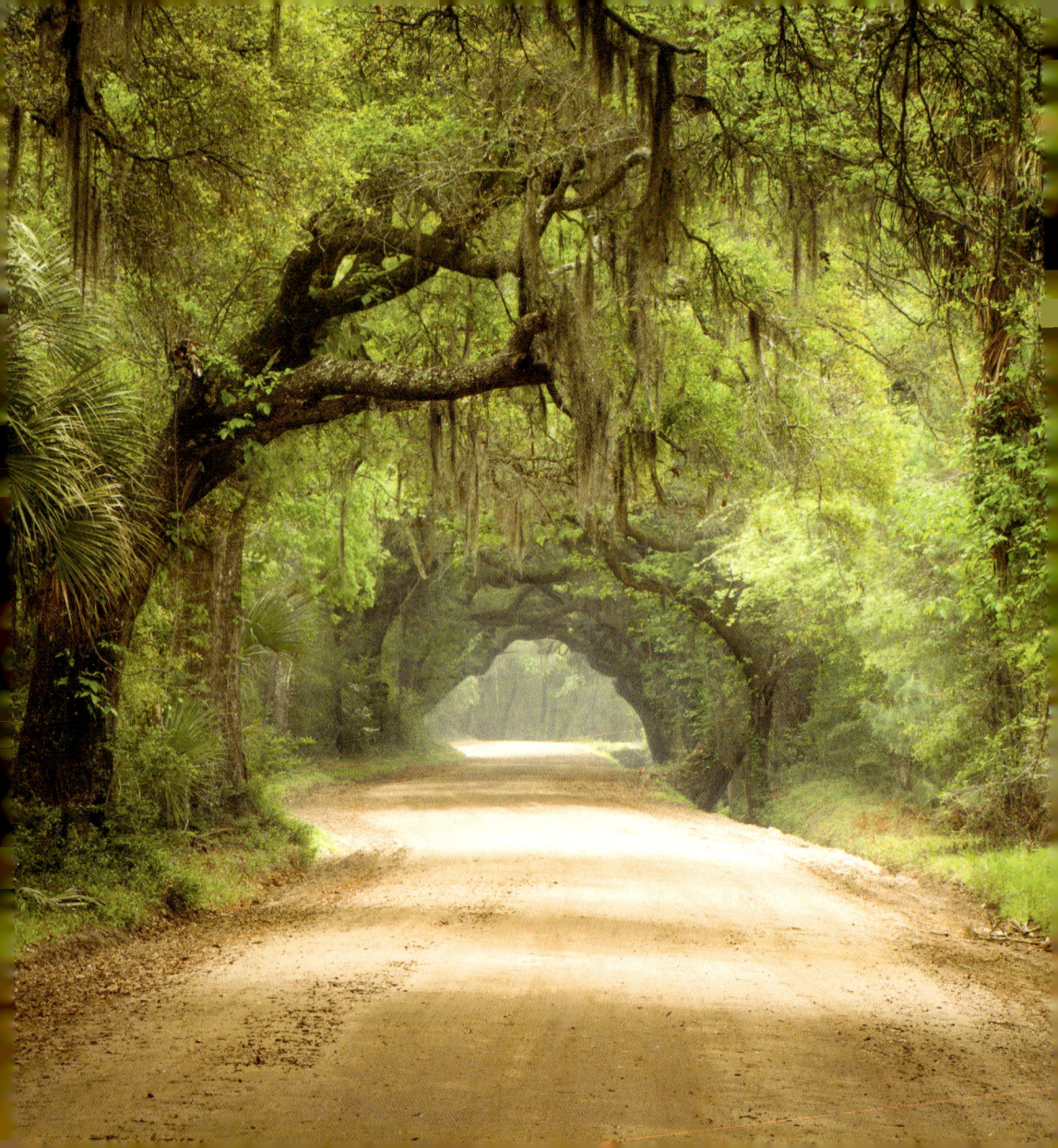

#4

Be your own advocate.

If you feel your safety is at risk, suspect an error or your medication is making you feel sick, speak up. To avoid infection, ask your care providers to wash their hands or put on gloves before treating you. When being transported or walking, take responsibility for making sure you don't slip and fall. Don't take risks. Wait for your caregivers to assist you.

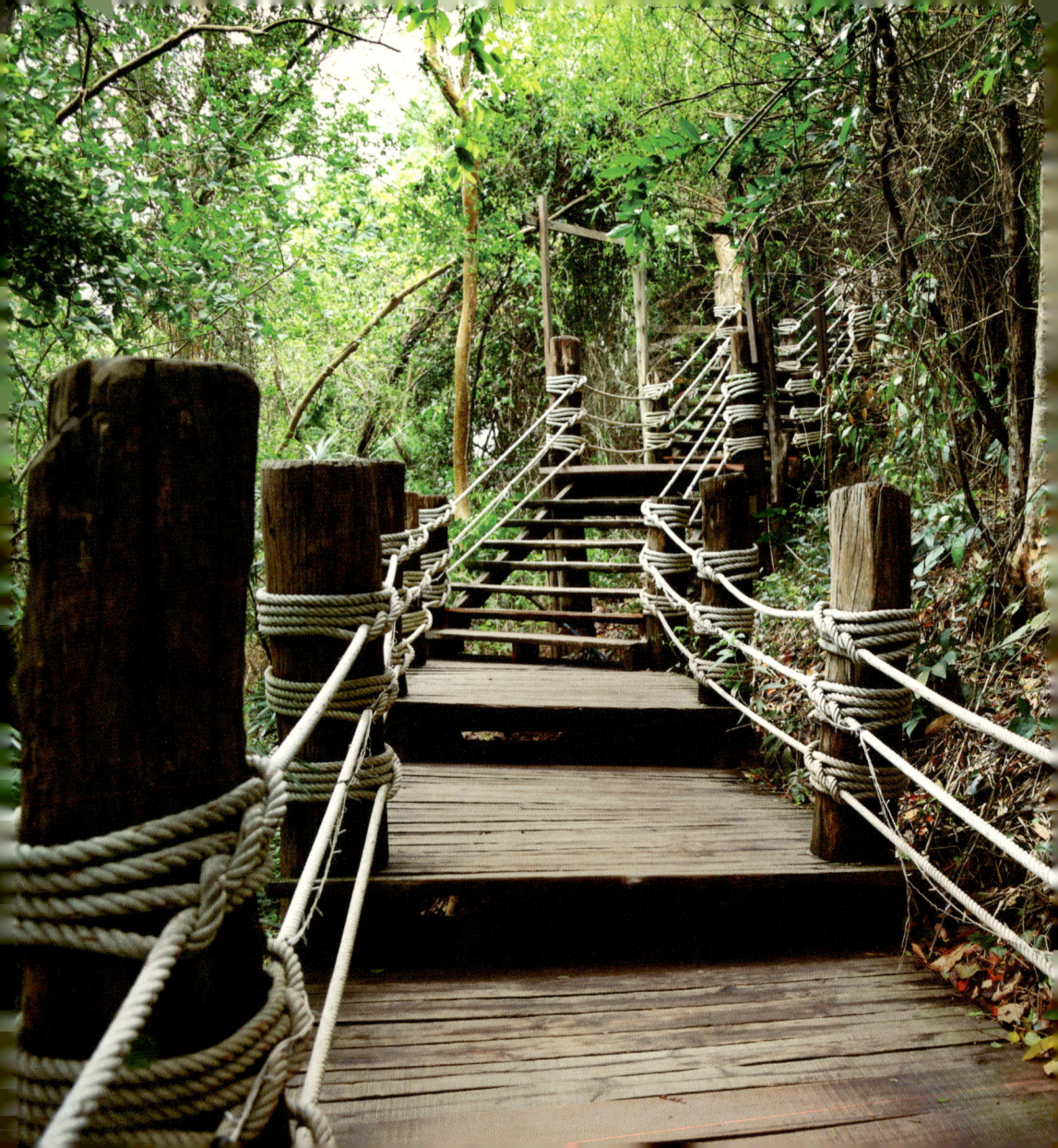

#5

Discuss health care directives.

Let your family and physicians know what actions and interventions should be taken on your behalf. Look into creating a Living Will and a Durable Power of Attorney for Health Care. Don't procrastinate. Get this done before leaving the hospital.

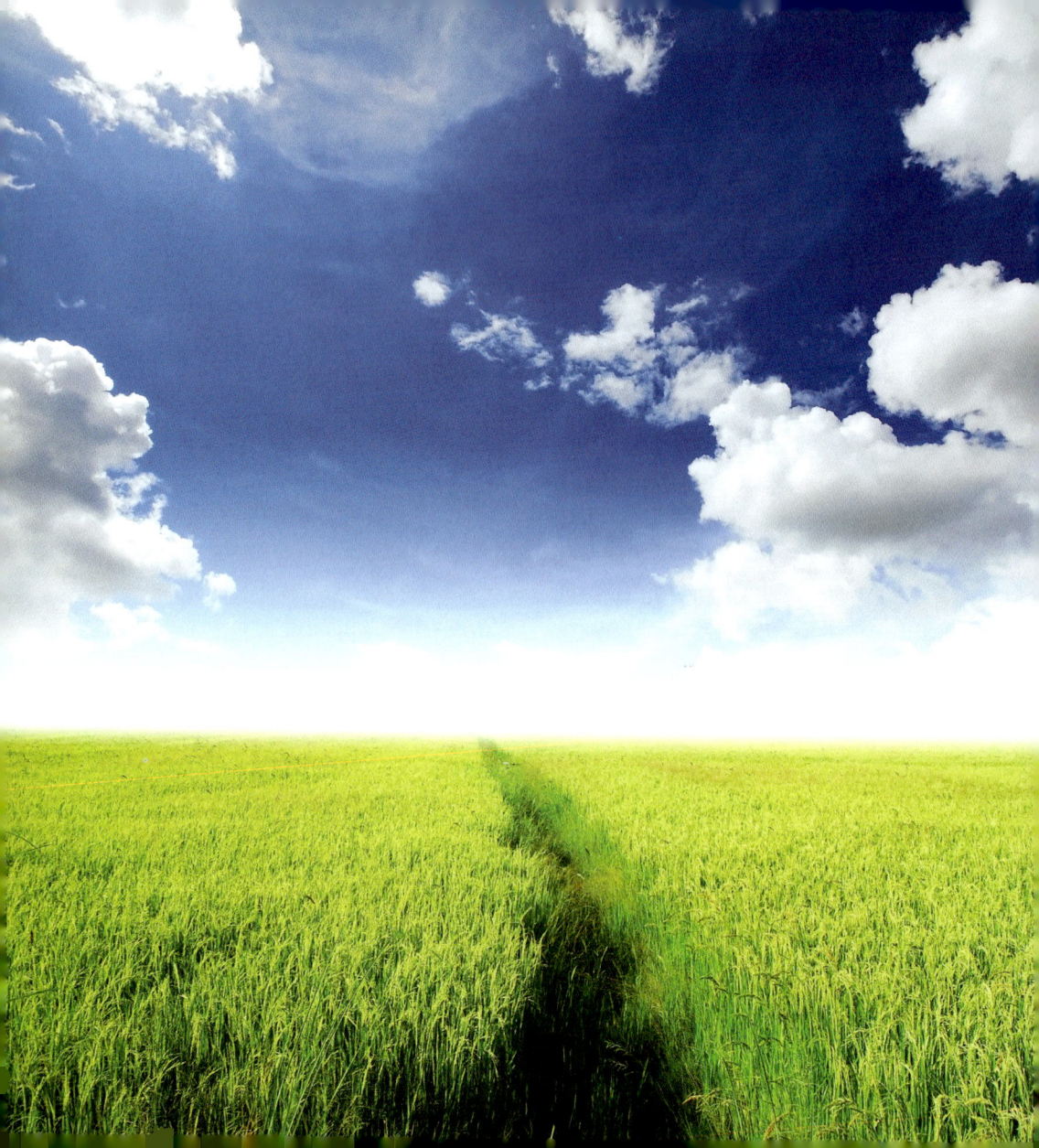

#6

Make your room One Positive Place.

Make your hospital room a place "For Positive People Only." Be selective about the television you watch and newspapers and magazines you read. Shift your focus to positive stories that are motivating, healing and a source of inspiration. Ask someone to put up positive pictures and encouraging words where you can see them. Ask your family, friends and caretakers to stay positive in your presence.

#7

Create Positive Relationships.

Be a creator not a critic. Establish good rapport with each member of your care-giving team, which includes everyone at the hospital as well as your family and friends. Working in health care today is an extremely challenging occupation and your caregivers are trying their best to create positive experiences for you. They could use some encouraging words from time to time. It can also be very stressful for your family and friends when they come to visit. Try to share some good news with them. It is in your best interest to create positive relationships with the people who enter your room. You have the power to bring out the best or worst in the people who care for you. Decide today that you are going to build better relationships with the people who are helping you. Caring for those who care for you will accelerate your healing process.

And when you are ready, *be a positive influence on other patients.* During World War II, a surprising discovery was made that can affect your recovery today. Because there were not enough nurses in post-operative care during the war, military patients were encouraged to help other military patients as soon as they started to recover. The result? Those patients did better and returned to duty faster.

Stephen Post, Ph.D., co-author of the book *"Why Good Things Happen to Good People"* said, "Since depression, anxiety, and stress involve a high degree of focus on the self, focusing on the needs of others literally helps shift our thinking. When you're experiencing compassion, benevolence, and kindness, they push aside the negative emotions. One of the best ways to overcome stress is to do something to help someone else."

During your stay in the hospital there is a good chance you are going to meet another patient or caregiver who needs an encouraging word or a smile. Everyone wins when you choose to be a positive influence on others. Give it a try. See if you feel better when you help someone else.

#8

Ask for help.

If you're in pain, need an extra blanket, help with meals or getting out of bed, ask for assistance. If it's too loud at night, ask someone to shut your door, ask for earplugs or a headset to listen to something soothing.

Be positive and specific when making requests and don't accept a vague response. "I'll try" or "As soon as possible" can mean anything. You may interpret that answer to imply your nurse will be back in 5 minutes, but your nurse might have a different time frame in mind. You can help your caregivers help you by being clear on what you need and why you need it.

Seeking and accepting the support of others is a critical part of your healing process. Too many patients don't ask for what they need because they don't want to bother their caregivers. If that negative thought ever enters your mind, remember what we just said in Positive Action Number 7. People feel better when they help others. Do your caregivers a favor and let them assist you.

It's also important for you to know that your hospital is a busy place and there are hundreds of patients in need of care. If you don't get what you need in the time that it was promised, be pleasantly persistent when following up. Your caregivers will appreciate your thoughtfulness.

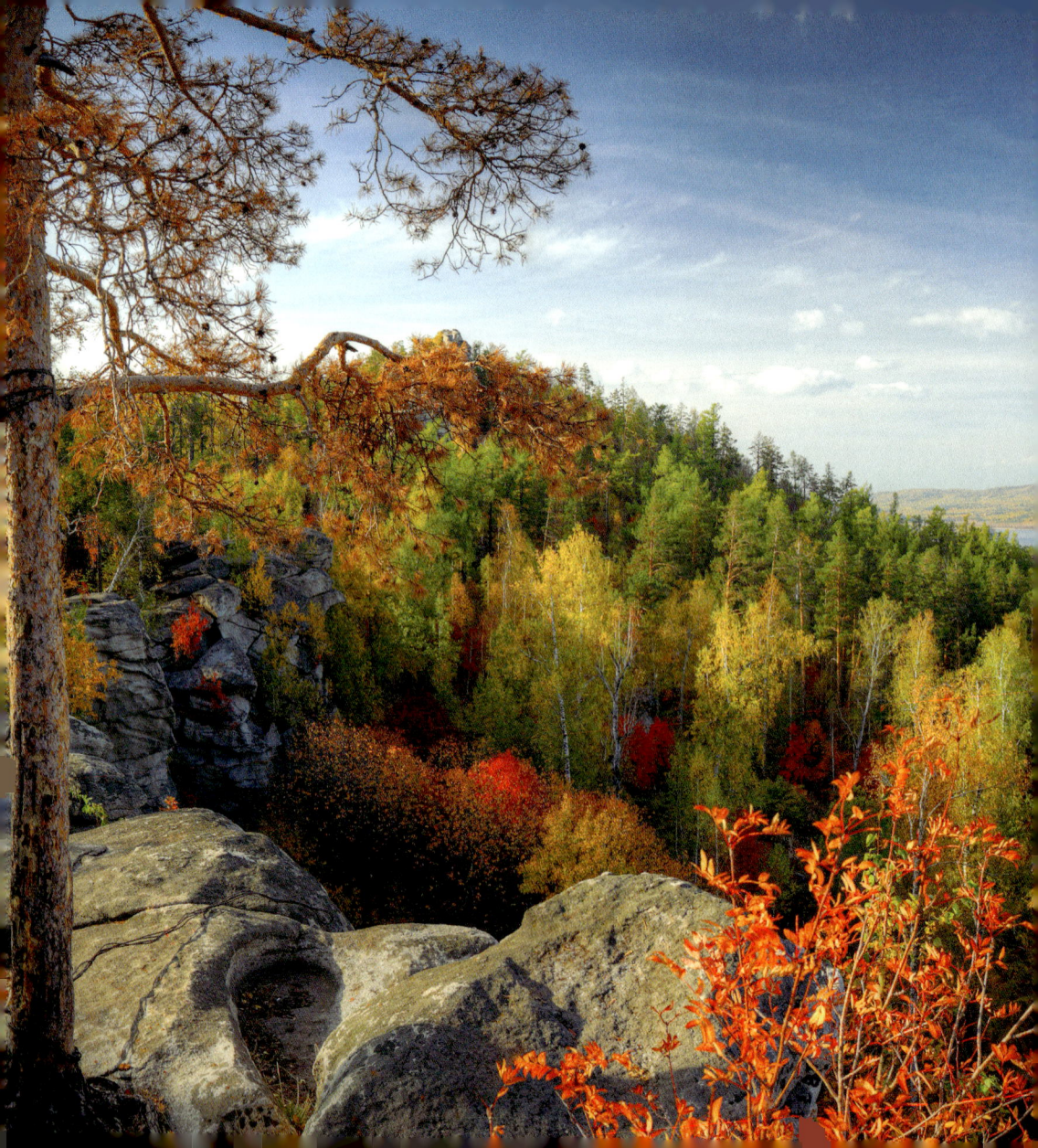

#9 Create inner peace.

Immerse yourself in activities you find relaxing. Read an uplifting book. Listen to calming music. Watch a favorite movie. Meditate. Reflect on the positive people in your life. Focus on feeling better. List all the things you are grateful for, identify your God-given talents and determine how you can use your strengths to serve others who are suffering.

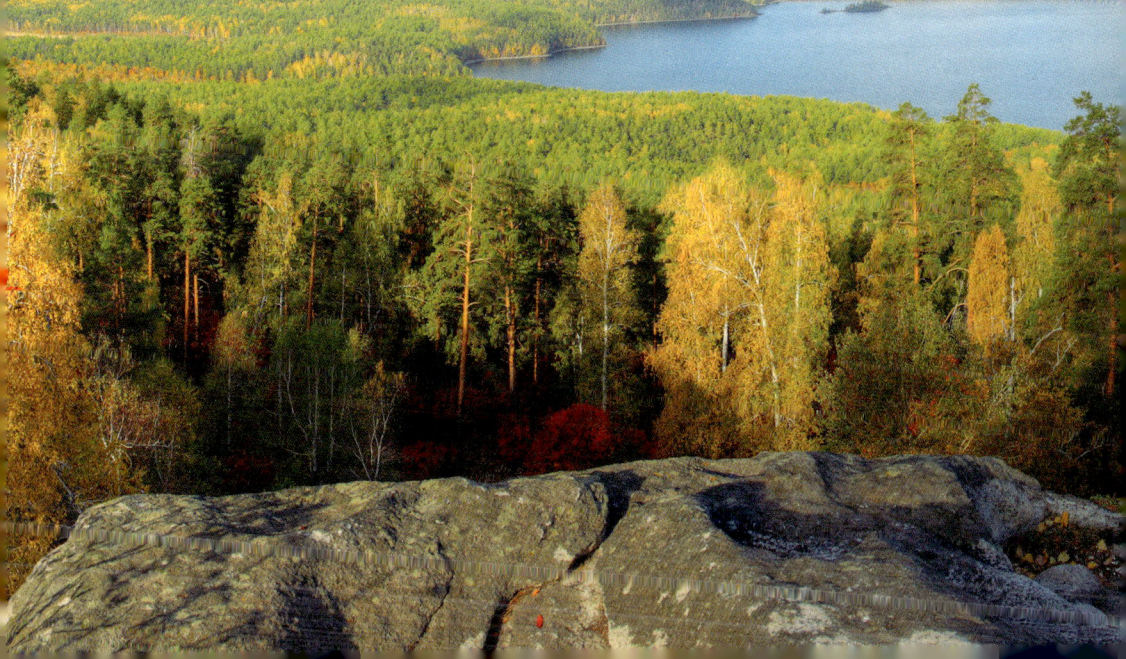

#10

Use humor to heal.

Learn to laugh at situations out of your control. Lighten the mood with caregivers and visitors. Tap into the benefits of laughter to give your mind and body a healthy boost. Find something to smile about. I know you don't always feel like smiling when you're in the hospital but, whenever possible, give someone a sincere smile. It will make both of you feel better.

The Meaning of a Smile

It costs nothing but it creates much.

It enriches those who receive it without impoverishing those who give it.

It happens in a flash and yet the memory of it sometimes lasts forever.

There are none so rich that they can get along without it,
and none so poor but are richer for its benefits.

It creates happiness in the home,
fosters goodwill in a business and is the countersign of friends.

It is rest to the weary, daylight to the discouraged, sunshine to the sad
and nature's best antidote for trouble, and yet it cannot be begged,
bought, borrowed or stolen; for it is something that is no earthly good
to anyone until it is given away.

So if in the course of the day your friends may be too tired to give you a smile,
then why don't you give them one of yours, because nobody needs a smile more
than those who have none left to give.

SMILE

Hal Roach, Irish Comedian

What positive actions can you take today?

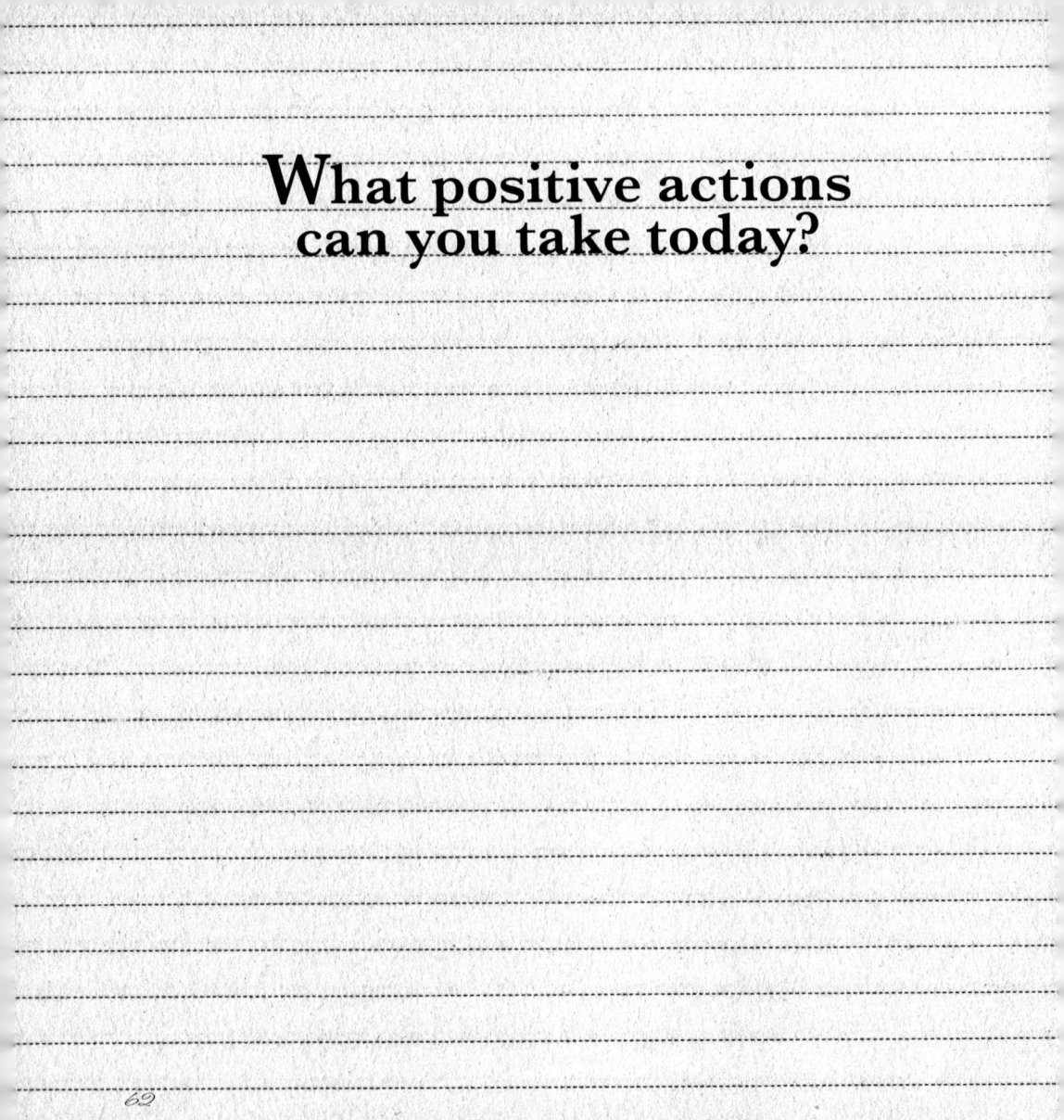

63

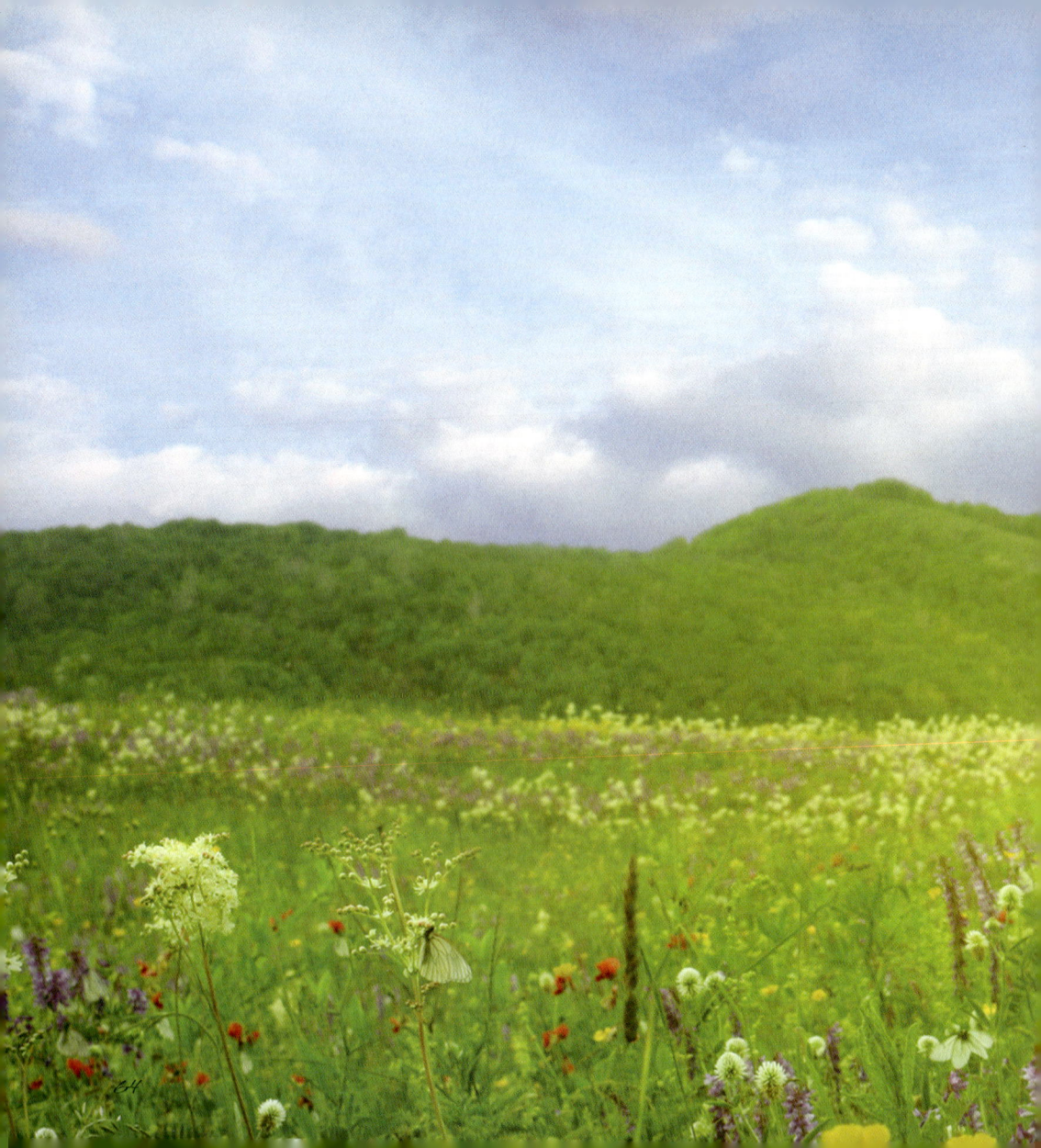

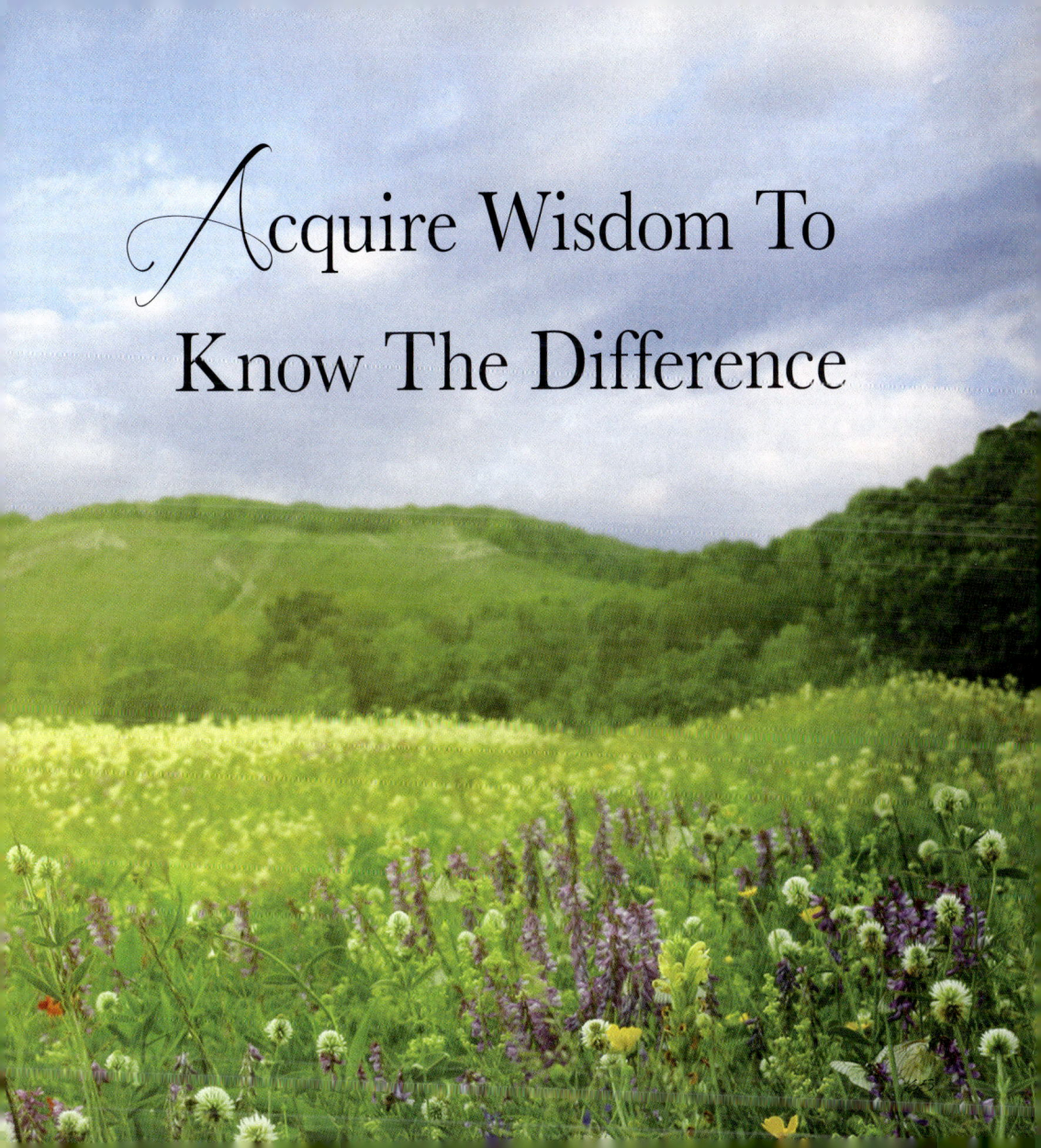

Acquire Wisdom To Know The Difference

Acquire Wisdom To Know The Difference

In the face of sudden or serious illness, we don't always know how to make the best decisions or what actions to take. In choosing whether to accept our circumstances or gather the strength to fight, how do we acquire "the wisdom to know the difference?"

Wisdom asks that we be present and attentive. It requires that we see and hear in the moment to discern "Our Truth."

When the diagnosis is serious, how long do you fight? How do you know when to roll up your sleeves and when to accept the grace of knowing you've done all you can? When family is involved, how can you find peace and confidence in your personal choices when they may be in conflict with the hopes of those you love?

How do you keep going when you're not clear about the path to take? How do you make decisions about something you've never done before? While pain and suffering often leave us with feelings of helplessness, isolation or defeat, it also opens opportunities for deep reflection. When we're facing what may seem like insurmountable problems, it helps if we can develop the spiritual guidance necessary to keep moving in a positive direction.

Whether you find spirituality in the pew of a Chapel, Temple or surrounded by nature, each of us can tap into a place to quiet our mind, follow our God or Higher Power and find the peace and confidence of knowing what direction will be the right path today. To acquire the wisdom to make good decisions, sometimes it requires us to slow down, take a deep breath and ask for guidance. It may be in the form of prayer, meditation or simply embracing the silence to listen to your inner guide. Remember *"The Serenity Prayer"* starts with "God grant me…" You are not alone.

"Wisdom is not a product of schooling but of the lifelong attempt to acquire it."

—Albert Einstein

Positive Questions for Hope and Healing

As you seek the wisdom to "know the difference" between the things you cannot change and the things you can, embark on a spiritual quest. Ask your God for insights to help you make positive choices. Be willing to trust the voice that guides you. When searching for answers, don't be afraid to ask difficult questions.

You can start seeking the wisdom to know the difference between what you should accept and what you can change while in the hospital and continue the process when you get home. Developing wisdom is a journey, not a destination.

Here are some questions for your reflection:

- What should I accept about my life now?

_____
_____
_____
_____

- How can I find peace in accepting what I cannot change?

_____
_____
_____
_____

Acquire Wisdom To Know The Difference

- How can I benefit by accepting what I can't change?

_____
_____
_____
_____

- What positive actions can I take to get better?

_____
_____
_____
_____

- What do I want to stop doing or start doing today?

_____
_____
_____
_____

- Where do I find the inner strength to fight for the best quality of life today?

_____
_____
_____
_____

Acquire Wisdom To Know The Difference

- *Based on the facts of my diagnosis, what are my best options?*

_____
_____
_____
_____

- *What is the purpose for the rest of my life?*

_____
_____
_____
_____

- What legacy do I want to leave for my family and friends?

_____
_____
_____
_____

- What can I do to show my love for the most important people in my life?

_____
_____
_____
_____

Acquire Wisdom To Know The Difference

- How can I let go of my anger?

_____
_____
_____
_____

- Who needs my forgiveness?

_____
_____
_____
_____

- *How* will I benefit by forgiving others?

_____
_____
_____
_____

- *How* can I find the confidence to reassure my family about my choices?

_____
_____
_____
_____

- **How will I know when it's time to consider a different path?**

_____
_____
_____
_____

- **How can I develop the wisdom to know what can and cannot be changed?**

_____
_____
_____
_____

- What can I do to turn my problems into a positive experience?

_____
_____
_____
_____

- How can I make my situation better?

_____
_____
_____
_____

- How can I become more optimistic?

_____
_____
_____
_____

- Who can I help today?

_____
_____
_____
_____

- *How can I learn to live one day at a time?*

  _____
  _____
  _____
  _____

- *Which choices will lead me to serenity?*

  _____
  _____
  _____
  _____

- What are the highest priorities in my life right now?

_____
_____
_____
_____

- What can I do to **Strive to Thrive Today?**

_____
_____
_____
_____

Notes:

Acquire Wisdom To Know The Difference

Notes:

Notes:

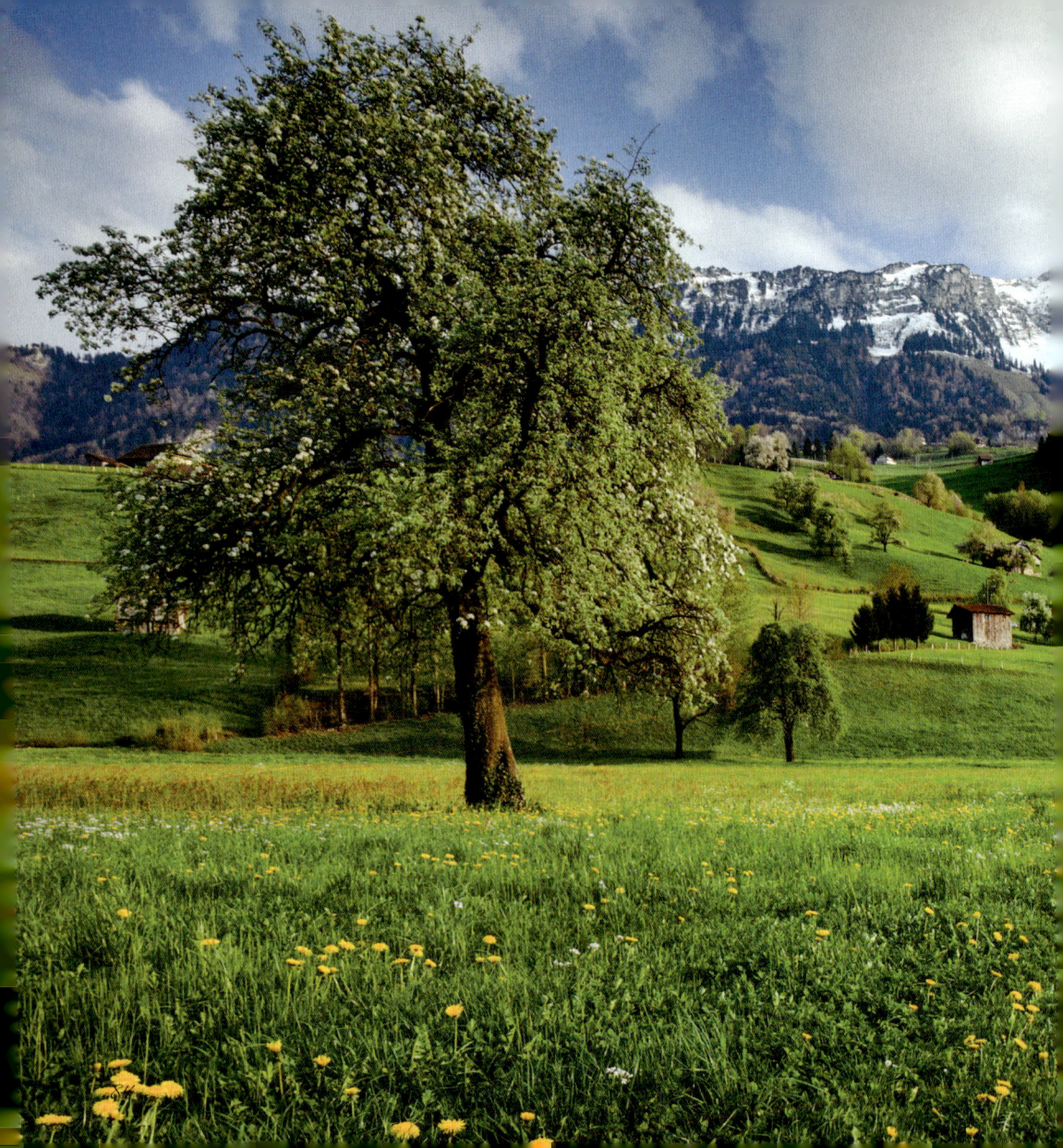

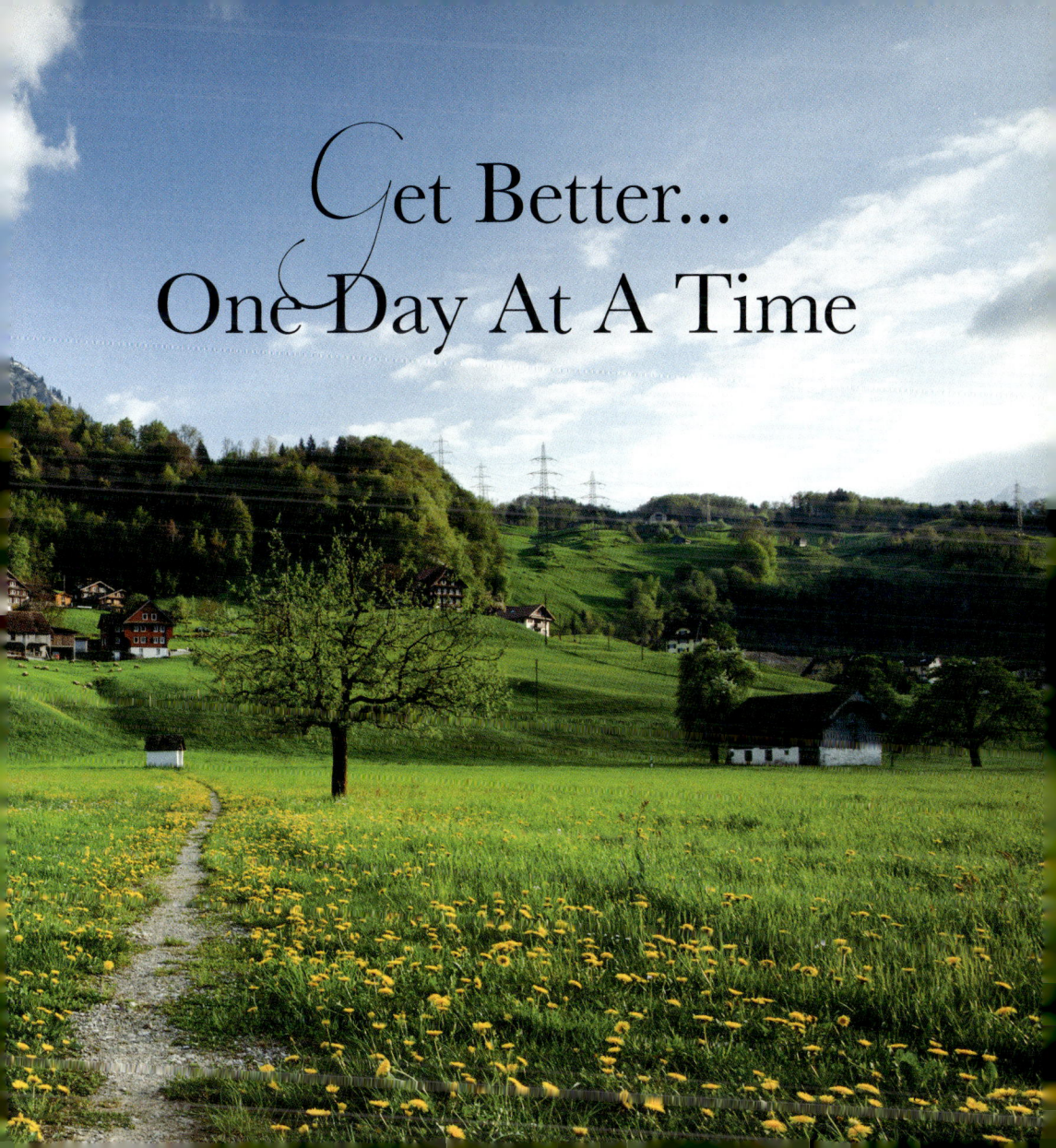

Get Better...
One Day At A Time

Get Better...One Day At A Time

In the first few days after leaving the hospital, I found it hard to stay focused on answering the questions I just shared with you. While my body was healing, there was something missing from my mental recovery. Then one day, I realized I needed to give myself a present—one that couldn't be bought in a store or on the Internet. No family member or friend could supply what I needed to receive. The gift I required was giving myself permission to live in the present, one day at a time...one moment at a time.

I knew the real problem was not in my back, but in my approach to my circumstances. I didn't have control of my thoughts. My mind bounced between worrying about the future to regretting lost opportunities in the past. I wasn't sure if yesterday or tomorrow would win the battle for the most time on my mind, but the loser was always the same—me.

When I lived in the past, I felt a sense of loss about not being able to do what I had previously done. When I pondered the future, I could not see a scenario that would make the rest of my life better. If I wanted to thrive, I had to learn to live in the moment and not waste time thinking negatively about yesterday or tomorrow.

Fortunately, I had been teaching positive seminars since the late 1970s. I knew that negative thoughts generate fears and doubts and that when I'm afraid, my focus narrows and all I can see are problems outside of my control. I was aware that fear could become an enemy that immobilizes and blinds me to positive possibilities. I also knew I needed to stop worrying. However, there is a big gap between knowing what to do and actually doing it.

Committing to live in the present moment is not easy, but it is a gift worth giving yourself. I guess that's why it's called the PRESENT. Making the commitment to stay positive and live one day at a time, in spite of your fears, is the only way to thrive.

...the moment one definitely commits oneself, then Providence moves too. All sorts of things occur to help one that would never otherwise have occurred...I learned a deep respect for one of Goethe's couplets: Whatever you can do or dream you can, begin it. Boldness has genius, power and magic in it!

–W. H. Murray *The Scottish Himalayan Expedition*

Take the 40-Day Positivity Challenge

When you are in the hospital, you have time to think about your life. During those moments of reflection, it's very common for someone to identify several positive changes they plan to make. Unfortunately, those good thoughts are treated more like New Year's resolutions. The intentions are admirable, but the commitment is weak. After a couple of days or weeks, it's back to your old habits.

Whether you decide to stay positive while accepting what you can't change and changing what you can is a personal choice. Everyone's situation is different. You may not be ready and that's OK. Just be honest with yourself. Accept your decision.

You may have family and friends that want you to do things differently but unless you are ready to make a commitment, it won't work. You will be back to your old habits in no time and it will be frustrating for everyone.

On the other hand, you may feel your illness or injury has been a wake-up call for you and you want to do something more meaningful with the time you have left. No matter how old or young you are, God has a purpose for your life; and, if you are reading this book, your purpose is not complete.

If you're ready, I invite you to do an experiment with me. For the next 40 days, I'd like you to make a commitment to being a more positive person. The challenge won't be easy, but I'm convinced that by the end of this 40-day experience, the purpose for the rest of your life will be clearer and you will be a happier, healthier person. The ability to thrive, in spite of your challenges, requires a consistently positive point of view.

Each morning, make a commitment to think and act in positive ways. Accept those things you can't change with a positive attitude, have the courage to change the things you can and ask God for help developing wisdom. Make a commitment to bring joy, peace and meaning into your life and the lives of those around you. Look for opportunities to use your strengths to lighten the load for others. Accentuate the positive in every conversation. Be a positive influence on the people who cross your path and teach those who are ready to do the same.

Get Better...One Day At A Time

Establish an ongoing practice of expressing gratitude to your family, friends and caregivers. Notice when someone is being helpful, kind and considerate and convey your appreciation. Send at least one thank you note to someone who has had a positive impact in your life and whenever possible, deliver that letter in person.

Remember…everybody makes somebody happy…for some it's when they enter a room and for others it's when they leave a room. Make sure you do your best to help others feel better when they are with you. You'll be surprised by how often you can bring out the best in yourself and others when your thoughts, words and actions are positive.

If a negative idea enters your mind at any time during the day, create 3 positive thoughts immediately. Rate yourself on the positivity scale every 4 hours and determine what positive actions you can take to achieve or maintain a positive point of view.

Don't wait until you feel motivated to do something positive. Base your actions today on your commitments, not your feelings. You cannot create positive change if you allow negative feelings to determine your direction.

When you leave the hospital, incorporate some ideas from the Positive Action Plan on pages 40-60 into your daily routine.

0	2	4	6	8	10
++ +++	++ ++−	++ +−−	++ −−−	+− −−−	−− −−−

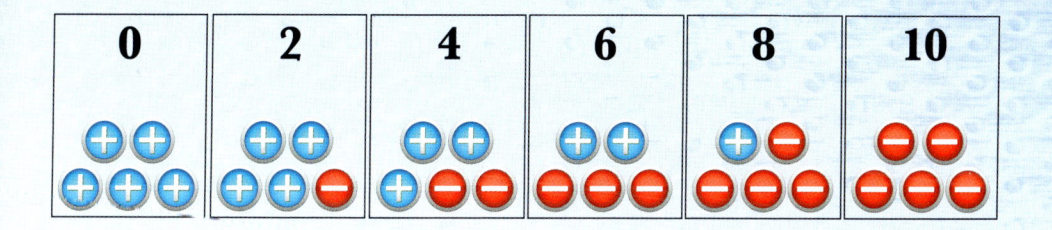

    0.................... Always Positive

    2.................... Mostly Positive

    4.................... A little more Positive than Negative

    6.................... A little more Negative than Positive

    8.................... Mostly Negative

    10.................... Always Negative

At the end of your day, right before you go to bed, reflect on what you did well and capture your positive insights in the 40 Day Challenge Journal at the back of this book. As you fall asleep, keep thinking about what you did to make your world a more positive place.

Repeat this process for the next 40 days.

NO EXCUSES!

One More Story

When I met Kyle Maynard, he changed my life for good. Kyle was born with arms that end at the elbows and legs near the knees. In spite of those limitations, Kyle played football in grammar school, wrestled for his high school team, set records in weightlifting, fought in mixed martial arts, wrote a best-selling book called *"No Excuses"* and most recently became the first man to crawl on his own to the summit of Mt. Kilimanjaro, the highest mountain in Africa.

Kyle was the keynote speaker at a convention I attended in California. I have heard some great speakers over the years, but no one has inspired me more than Kyle. His "No Excuses, Anything is Possible" talk was not unique. I've listened to those messages most of my adult life. I was impressed with his character and his ability to help me look differently at the obstacles in my life. In just 90 minutes, he gave me, and I believe all 2,000 people in the room, the strength to know that excuses would never be part of our lives again. I walked out of that convention center extremely impressed with Kyle; but more importantly, I felt better about myself. Given all his challenges, if Kyle could live with "no excuses," so could I…and so can you.

Later that evening, I had the pleasure of having dinner with Kyle. The only thing more amazing than hearing him add to his story was watching him eat, drink and autograph his book with his elbows. I don't know how many hours Kyle has spent learning to do things I take for granted every day. What I do know is that you and I can live happier, healthier, more meaningful lives by following his example. I'm not just talking about living with a "No Excuses" attitude. While that's important, it's not enough. What makes Kyle so amazing is that he has dedicated his life to maximizing his God-given talents and using those strengths to serve others in an extraordinary way. He has made a commitment to thrive, not merely survive, in spite of the obstacles in his life.

Are you ready to take positive action today despite your injury or illness…perhaps even changing the lives of others you encounter? I hope you will make a commitment to stay positive and **Strive to Thrive Today!** Remember the lessons of *"The Serenity Prayer"*…God will grant you the ability to accept the things you cannot change, have the courage to change the things you can and have the wisdom to know the difference.

Stay Positive

Even in the midst of pain and loss, there is still beauty in our lives. We just need to see it or create it. Optimism is an empowering virtue. When we consciously choose to focus on the good, the positive impact radiates to all facets of our physical, emotional, spiritual, and social well-being. The results and rewards are energizing.

When we focus on the positive, we no longer feel like victims. We can begin to create joy for ourselves and others. Our attitude and behavior energizes and encourages the people around us. Our efforts help others to thrive.

Too many patients set their goals for recovery too low. Fixing the problem that put you in the hospital is important, but it's not the end of the journey, it's only the beginning. Regardless of the obstacles in your path, you were born to thrive not just survive.

Staying positive and making an effort to thrive is a continuous process and a daily discipline for me. I'm not trying to be perfect anymore. Each day, I wake up and ask God for the strength to stay positive, accept what I can't change, change what I can and have the wisdom to know the difference, not for the rest of my life but just for today. I don't want to worry about tomorrow or get discouraged by what I didn't do yesterday. I want to make my world a more positive place for my family and friends. I want to live and thrive one day at a time. I want the same thing for you.

Thrive or Survive...
It's Your Choice

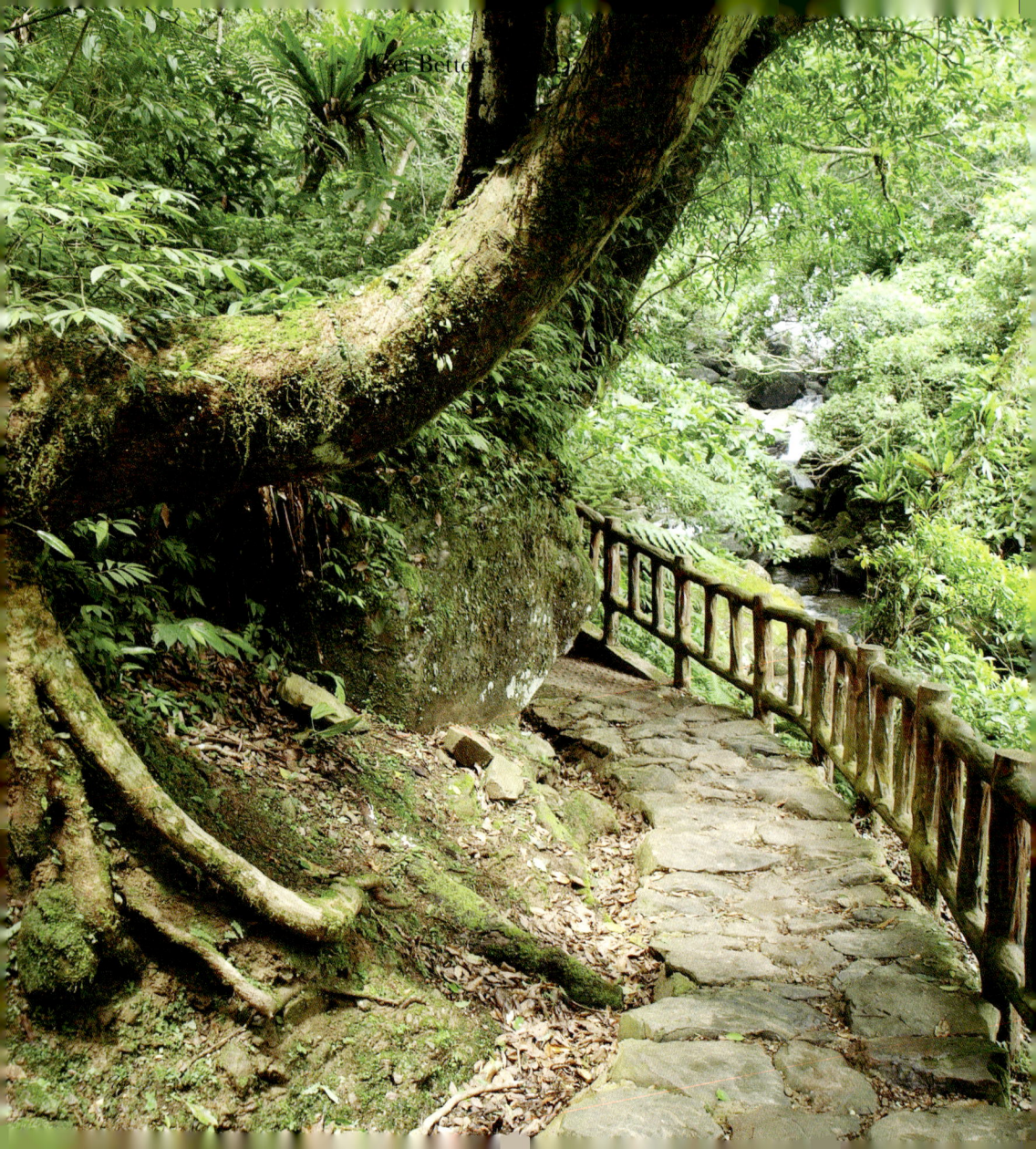

Are you ready to
Stay Positive
&
Strive to Thrive Today?

If your answer is yes, please sign your name below and join me in the 40 Day Positivity Challenge. The Challenge asks you to put the concepts from this book into **ACTION** until they become a habit. By committing to stay positive and thrive, every day for the next 40 days, you will be making the choice to maximize your health and flourish during the highs and lows of life.

Ready? Let's Get Better…Together!

Review pages 88-91, and let's get started.

_____	*Bill Durkin*
Sign Your Name	Bill Durkin

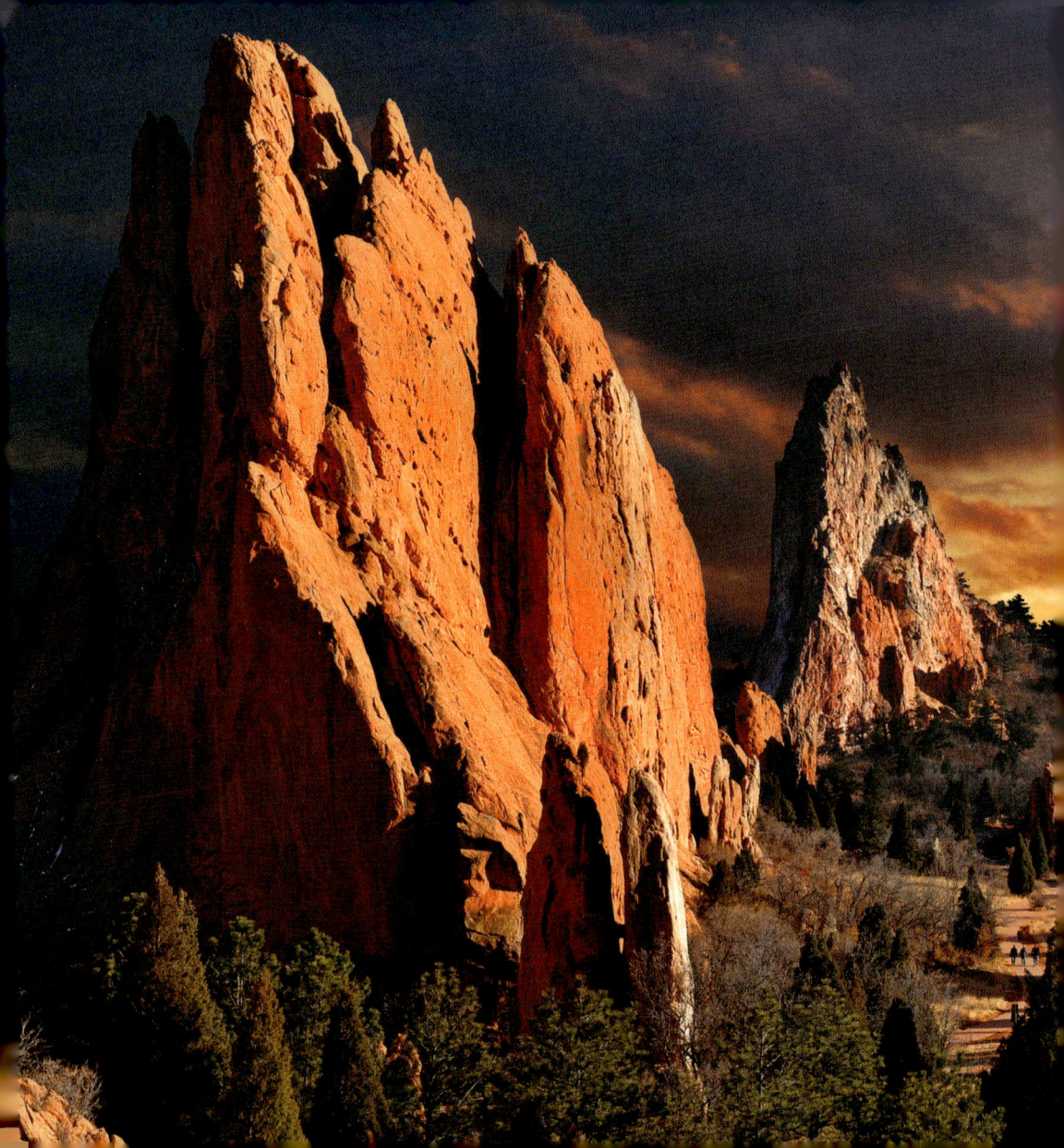

40 Day Challenge Journal

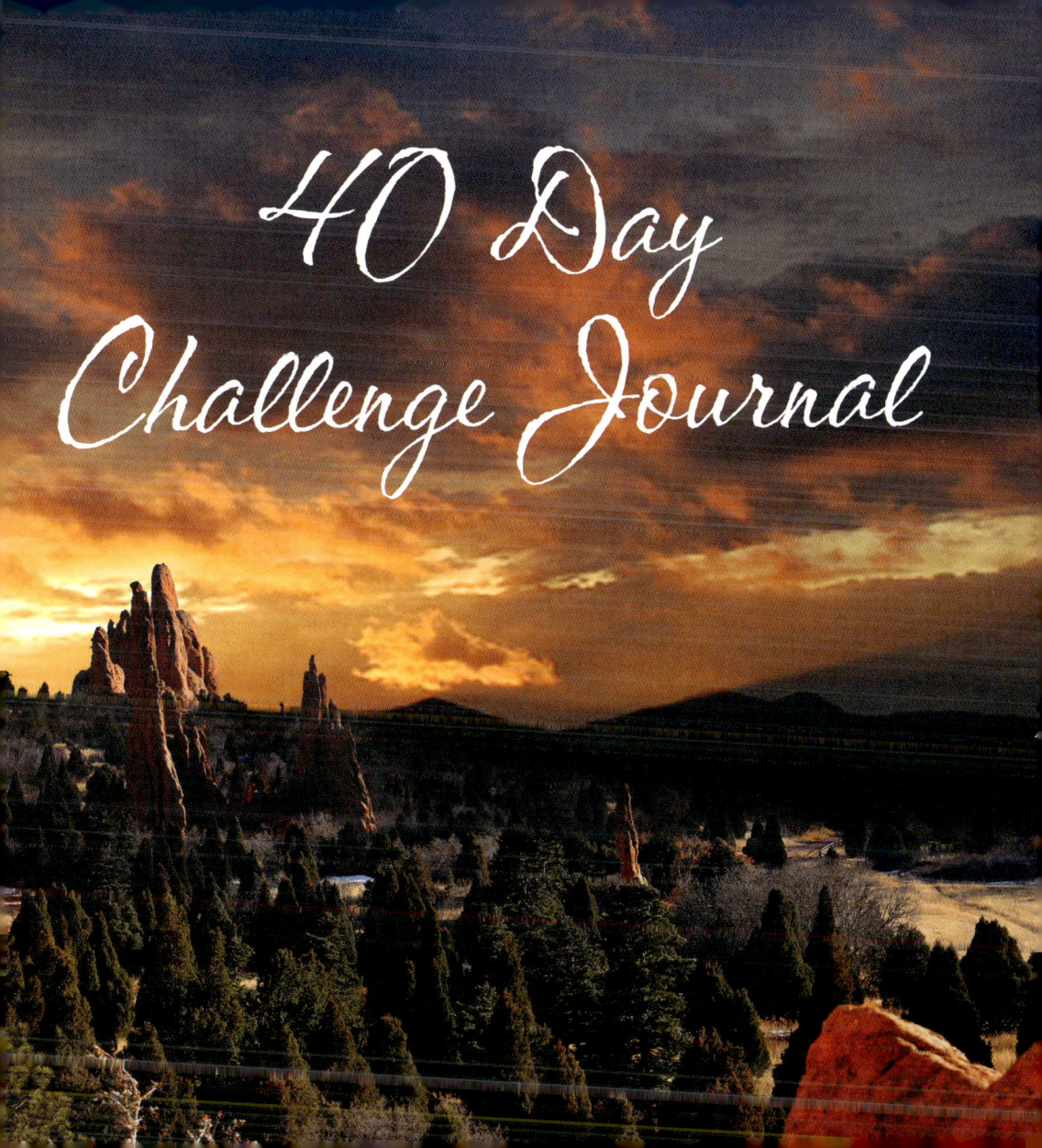

Day 1

"There is very little difference in people, but that little difference makes a big difference. The little difference is attitude."
-W. Clement Stone

Day 2

"All our dreams can come true,
if we have the courage to pursue them."
-Walt Disney

Day 3

"If you don't like something, change it.
If you can't change it, change your attitude."
-Maya Angelou

Day 4

*"We are what we repeatedly do.
Excellence, then, is not an act, but a habit."
-Aristotle*

Day 5

"Gratitude is the key to happiness."
-C.S. Lewis

Day 6

"Every problem has a gift for you in its hands."
-Richard Bach

Day 7

"It takes a lot of courage to show your dreams to someone else."
—Erma Bombeck

Day 8

"Live so that when your children think of fairness, caring, and integrity, they think of you."
—H. Jackson Brown, Jr.

Day 9

"To keep the body in good health is a duty...otherwise we shall not be able to keep our mind strong and clear."
-Buddha

Day 10

"A man is but the product of his thoughts – what he thinks, he becomes."
— Mahatma Gandhi

Day 11

"Worry never robs tomorrow of its sorrow, it only saps today of its joy."
—Leo Buscaglia

Day 12

"A pessimist sees the difficulty in every opportunity; an optimist sees the opportunity in every difficulty."
 —Winston Churchill

Day 13

"A year from now, you may wish you had started today."
-Karen Lamb

Day 14

"You must do the thing you think you cannot do."
— Eleanor Roosevelt

Day 15

"Change your thoughts, and you change your world."
—Norman Vincent Peale

Day 16

"The best way to predict the future is to create it."
— Peter F. Drucker

Day 17

"Kind words can be short and easy to speak, but their echoes are truly endless."
−Mother Teresa

Day 18

"The best thing to give to your enemy is forgiveness, to your child, a good example."
—Benjamin Franklin

Day 19

"Happiness is an attitude. We either make ourselves miserable, or happy and strong. The amount of work is the same."
-Francesca Reigler

Day 20

"The future belongs to those who believe in the beauty of their dreams."
—Benjamin Franklin

Day 21

"If you realized how powerful your thoughts are, you would never think a negative thought."
—Peace Pilgrim

Day 22

"Even if you are on the right track,
you'll get run over if you just sit there."
-Will Rogers

Day 23

"Learn to get in touch with the silence within yourself and know that everything in life has a purpose."
-Elisabeth Kübler-Ross

Day 24

"Not all of us can do great things.
But we can do small things with great love."
-Mother Teresa

Day 25

"How wonderful it is that nobody need wait a single moment before starting to improve the world."
-Anne Frank

Day 26

"Write it on your heart that every day is the best day in the year."
—Ralph Waldo Emerson

Day 27

"It takes a great deal of courage to stand up to your enemies, but even more to stand up to your friends."
-J. K. Rowling

Day 28

"Never give up, for that is just the place and time that the tide will turn."
—Harriet Beecher Stowe

Day 29

"Everybody can be great...because anybody can serve."
-Martin Luther King

Day 30

"Do your best and let God do the rest."
—Dr. Ben Carson

Day 31

"There is nothing wrong with going down.
It's staying down that's wrong."
-Muhammad Ali

Day 32

"I know God will never give me anything I can't handle. I just wish He didn't trust me so much."
— Mother Teresa

Day 33

"Obstacles are those frightful things you see when you take your eyes off your goal."
-Henry Ford

Day 34

"The greatest discovery of my generation is that a human being can alter his life by altering his attitude of mind."
—William James

Day 35

"Pessimism is a waste of time."
-Norma Cousins

Day 36

"There is a way to do it better. Find it."
—Thomas Edison

Day 37

"Don't let what you cannot do interfere with what you can do."
    -John R. Wooden

Day 38

"I am not afraid... I was born to do this."
  — Joan of Arc

Day 39

"I don't know the key to success,
but the key to failure is trying to please everybody."
-Bill Cosby

Day 40

"Go confidently in the direction of your dreams.
Live the life you have imagined."
-Henry David Thoreau

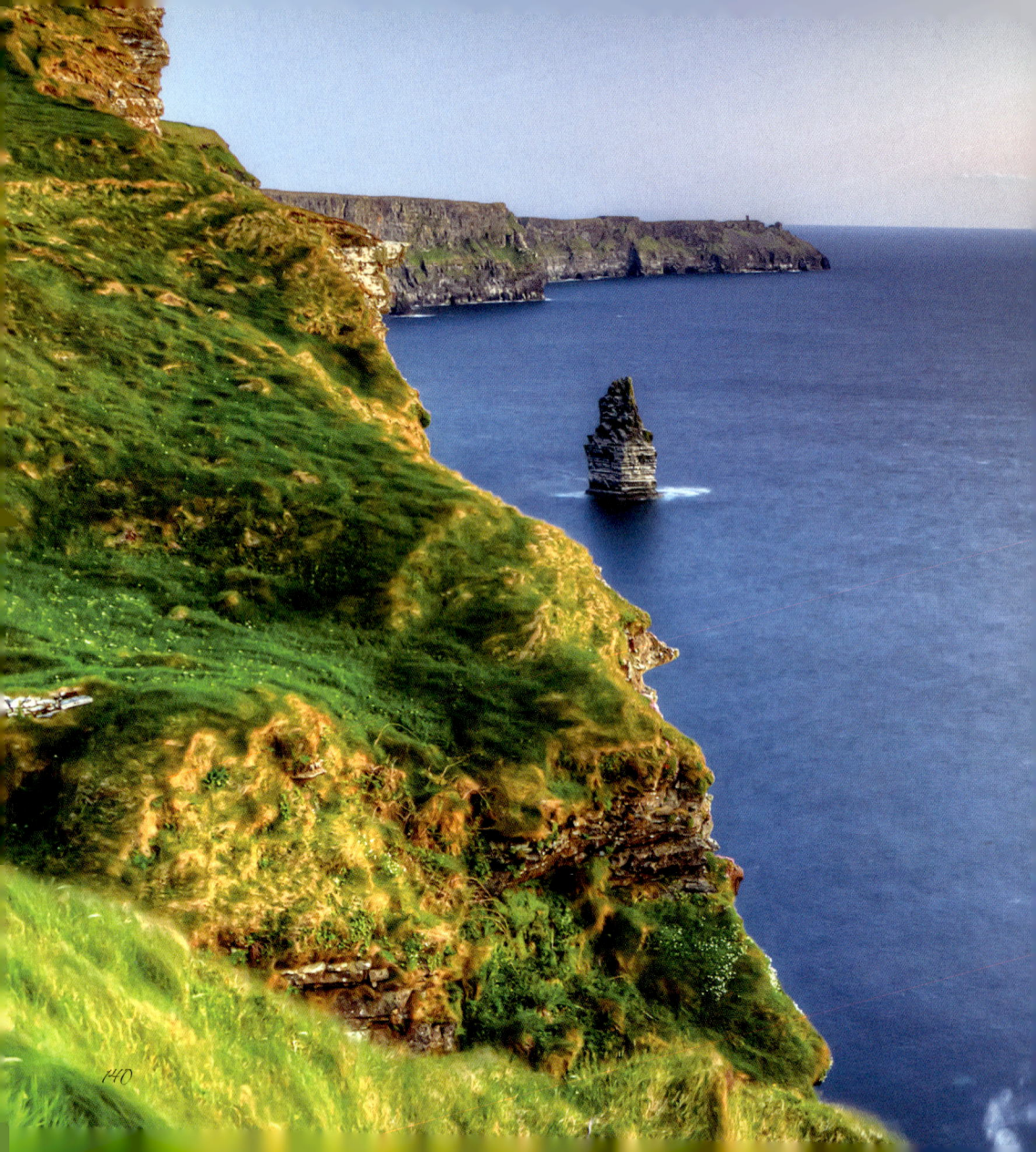

I believe that sharing positive stories is one of the most important things we can do to motivate and inspire others to be positive and thrive.

As you go through your 40 Day Positivity Challenge and apply the concepts from this book, please tell me what's working well for you. I will post the information on our website. www.strivetothrivetoday.com

Send your story to stories@strivetothrivetoday.com.

Thank you for your commitment to helping yourself and others **Strive to Thrive Today.**

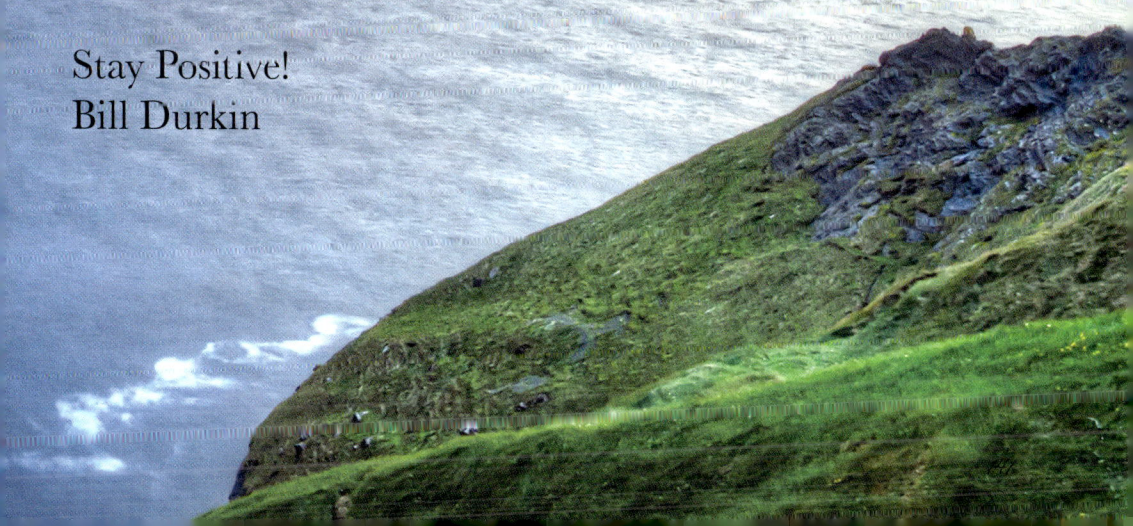

Stay Positive!
Bill Durkin

About the Author

Bill Durkin is an international speaker, consultant and coach. He is also founder of *One Positive Place*, a firm he started to help patients, family members and caregivers stay positive and thrive while in and out of the hospital. For more than 30 years, Bill has been providing education and encouragement to individuals around the world.

He has been President of two non-profit boards (Stauros USA & The National Speakers Association-Illinois Chapter), Chairman of the Corporate Network for the Association of Corporate Growth in Chicago, and has served as an Alderman in Darien, Illinois.

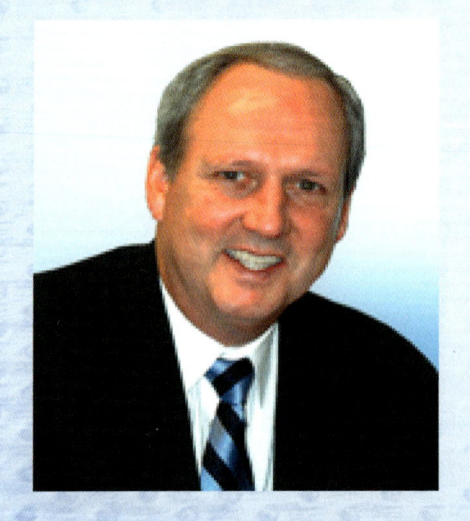

Bill was selected to the International Who's Who of Entrepreneurs and was honored with the prestigious Gold Leaf Award from Metropolitan Family Services in recognition of his volunteer work to strengthen families and communities.

He began his speaking career working closely with W. Clement Stone, author of *"Success Through a Positive Mental Attitude."* Bill taught his positive programs at corporations and correctional facilities around the country. He later served as a consultant and independent instructor for the Forum Corporation, which helps senior leaders execute innovative, people-driven solutions that accelerate business growth, corporate change and overall performance.

He has been recognized as a Certified Speaking Professional (CSP), a designation given to less than 10 percent of the speakers who belong to the National Speakers Association and the International Federation of Professional Speakers.

Bill lives with his wife and two sons in Darien, Illinois.

He presents regularly at conferences, corporations and association meetings. If you are interested in having Bill speak to your group, you can contact him at billdurkin@billdurkin.com or visit his website www.billdurkin.com to learn more about his speeches and seminars.